MICHEL TOWNSE

From
FEAR To
Freedom

When All Appears Lost,
A Way Will Be Found:
One Woman's Inspirational
Healing Journey To Freedom.

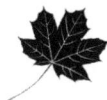

MAPLE
PUBLISHERS

From Fear To Freedom

Author: Michelle Townsend

Copyright © Michelle Townsend (2024)

The right of Michelle Townsend to be identified as author of this work has been asserted by the author in accordance with section 77 and 78 of the Copyright, Designs and Patents Act 1988.

First Published in 2024

ISBN 978-1-83538-057-4 (Paperback)
    978-1-83538-059-8 (E-Book)
    978-1-83538-058-1 (Hardback)

Book cover design and Book layout by:
    White Magic Studios
    www.whitemagicstudios.co.uk

Published by:
    Maple Publishers
    Fairbourne Drive, Atterbury,
    Milton Keynes,
    MK10 9RG, UK
    www.maplepublishers.com

In memory of my dear friend Lin.

Without you, this journey would not have been possible.

You helped me channel my 'inner Lin' just when I needed it most - never giving up.

For Mike, who changed my life forever.

For Karl, my rock.

Contents

Introduction .... *Page 7*

Author's Note .... *Page 13*

PART I: JOURNEY THROUGH DIS-EASE

Chapter 1 – Inner Child Programs... .... Page 17

Chapter 2 – Fitting In .... Page 29

Chapter 3 – Music was My First Love .... Page 41

Chapter 4 – M301! Here We Come .... Page 53

Chapter 5 – Momma World .... Page 59

Chapter 6 – Starting to Notice the Effects .... Page 71

Chapter 7 – Breaking Point! Journey to Hypnosis .... Page 87

PART II: UNDERSTANDING THE MIND

Chapter 8 – Hypnotherapy to the Rescue .... Page 103

Chapter 9 – Dear Diary .... Page 117

Chapter 10 – Best Decision Day .... Page 139

Chapter 11 – Challenging Change .... Page 153

Chapter 12 – The Big C! .... Page 165

Chapter 13 – Trials and Treatments .... Page 181

Chapter 14 – Journeys and Roller Coasters .... Page 195

Chapter 15 – Trust ... Faith ... Belief .... Page 211

Chapter 16 – It's OK .... Page 219

PART III: THERAPIES TO THERAPIST

Chapter 17 – Time for a Change .... Page 239

Chapter 18 – Rod of Iron .... Page 247

Chapter 19 – Message from the Other Side .... Page 261

Chapter 20 – Becoming Who I Am .... Page 273

Chapter 21 – Learning to Flow .... Page 285

Chapter 22 – A Way Will Be Found .... Page 293

Epilogue .... Page 297

Acknowledgements .... Page 299

Suggested Reading .... Page 303

About the Author .... Page 305

Introduction

*'Only when we let go of the past can we move from
FEAR to FREEDOM.'*

~ Michelle Townsend

I often think back to that October day in 2007, where my life was about to change - that time when I couldn't live my life with freedom. The sheer adversity of being unable to live my life fully led to the writing of this book and the guidance contained in it.

This book has been picked up and put down many times over 15 years, on this roller-coaster-ride of adversity. The intention of sharing my story lies in the possibilities that working with the mind can create powerful change within our lives. That no matter what we are going through or experiencing, no matter what is being thrown at us, a change in perspective really can shift someone to a place that they never would have thought they could connect with! It was a powerful realisation for me!

Little did I realise that the story about to unfold before me would not only be a complete game changer, but could also help others to realise the power they have within them too. Part of me must have known that I could inspire people to seek answers around adversity, their experiences and understanding the world around them. As a therapist now, I enjoy sharing parts of my experiences, knowing that others can benefit from it too. I freely explain what I have come to understand and what I have learned through experiencing Electromagnetic Hypersensitivity (EHS) and Hodgkin's Lymphoma Cancer. In this book, I'm sharing my experiences of both journeys and how I walked through the associated adversities. A journey of preparation followed by practice!

After years of experiencing the ill-effects of EHS followed by Hodgkin's Lymphoma Cancer and being seriously ill, I turned to hypnotherapy to help with what I was about to encounter. EHS had been the preparation, cancer was now the powerful practice! Everything I had learned from EHS was now about to be put into use - BIG TIME! By using hypnotherapy, I overcame the difficulties, adversity and discomfort of the two dis-eases. I learned how to navigate my thoughts, feelings and responses through trial and error. I used the imbalance I was experiencing to create change. It was my catalyst. By using the power of my subconscious mind, I connected back into my higher self.

With the increase of cancer cases rising and the rollout of more man-made electromagnetic waves across the earth (such as 5G), my teaching memoir aims to be a turning point in thought; fostering an awareness that thought 'can' change reality. It 'can' change the outcome of what seems like an impossible situation. It is a story about 'trust, faith and belief'. EHS isn't really an illness many people know about. In fact, my doctors were totally bemused by it. They never really believed me! I had researched and realised it was EHS that I was experiencing. I would find myself explaining my condition to others, only to be looked at as though I was out of my mind! People treated me as though I was some kind of alien from out of space! EHS is a highly controversial diagnosis, little is understood about it - it's pushed under the carpet, so to speak.

Electromagnetic Hypersensitivity has, in fact, been around for years. It is otherwise known as 'Microwave sickness', which first appeared in 1974 when the military started using man-made 'radiofrequency (RF)'. EHS rose to a new level in the 1990s, with the introduction of mobile phones and then later Wi-Fi. Some people experience minor symptoms, others severe and totally debilitating. With the increase of 5G, the electromagnetic frequencies (EMFs) are being taken to another level, with more people experiencing effects, some not even realising what it is. This book offers help and guidance regarding perspective. If we can change our perspective and maintain a positive mindset, then anything is possible.

There was also the question of whether EHS caused the cancer that followed. I had to change my thoughts around this. I had to maintain a clear image within my mind. I changed my perspective, my belief, choosing to not focus on diagnoses but instead focus on healing, seeing EMFs as a sea of *'energy'* sending healing. This allowed me to continue living my life symptom-free.

We are capable of much more than we could ever realise! If what we think creates our reality and our future, could we choose our thoughts better? Change our responses? Make a commitment to ourselves to direct our thoughts to create a future the way we truly want it? No matter what we are faced with, we can create powerful change and overcome the things that we believed we couldn't or even seemed impossible. Learning the amazing power of my subconscious mind would prove to be one of the best turning points in my life, far outreaching anything I could have ever imagined. It was extremely powerful and indeed, would save my life. If I had not ventured down the route of the mind and hypnotherapy, I probably wouldn't be here writing these words now; it could have been a very different story.

When we switch on to the idea that we are in control of our own life and how we direct it - that we are not necessarily the person who has been handed the bad card in life - things can change in an instant! We start to see life from a different perspective.

When we release that *self-pity*, that *woe is me*, that *nothing goes right for me*, and we change it to ... *'What's this showing me? What can I learn from this? How can I respond differently to create what I really want?'*... things change for the better!

We have a choice in any moment on how to respond to any situation. For the most part, these responses are automatic, learned from our past experiences, our peers, parents and teachers. So, what if we just stop? Acknowledge that we do have a choice in that moment and start to choose how we will respond to create a different reality? Why do we take reality as gospel? Can we look at reality in a different way?

The main part of my story began somewhere around 2002, a time when the physical discomfort started to kick in, albeit subtle at first, following through to real trauma. But how had I got here? How did I end up experiencing such physical pain? Had my outlook on life been wrong all along? What had I done or experienced to get me to this point? Initially, I kept believing that the reality in front of me was true. I can see it, I can feel it, so it must be true! It's happening to me, so why wouldn't it be true? As time moved on, I started to question life; I mean really question life. My approach completely changed. I started to see through the reality. I became aware of it in a very different way. ***Energy!*** The physical discomfort I was experiencing was about to train my brain into something that would change my life forever. It was, in fact, a blessing! The question was, had my experiences through life, right the way back from childhood, impacted me in some way? Had those experiences been responsible for the way I reacted, responded, ventured through life each step of the way? All these questions were just popping up in front of me, creating a thirst for deeper understanding. If I could understand why, would that help change things? Or on the flip side, do we really need to understand why?

This book is divided into three parts: **Part I: 'Journey Through Dis-ease.'** Here we journey through my early years and the way in which those early experiences demonstrated how the mind creates beliefs within us that can transcend and manifest into illness as we move through life. I share how I now understand the old thought patterns and beliefs that led to the adversity I experienced as I moved into my 30s.

Part II: 'Understanding the Mind.' I share the journey that led to *breaking point*, that point where enough was enough. The sheer adversity. Life was falling apart around me. Here I discovered the saviour - hypnotherapy. Adversity can be changed into a blessing; a blessing of healing that transforms beliefs, responses, reality - creating a very deep understanding of the mind - how powerful using the mind to heal the body can be. Literally, moving *'from fear to freedom!'*

Part III: 'Therapies to Therapist.' I was so grateful I had survived those journeys of painful adversity. I accepted them wholeheartedly but I wanted a change, needed a change; so, I took what I had learned and used it to develop myself into a therapist, ready to share my journey to help people - just like I have written this book that you now hold in your hands. I knew I could do it - after all, I had been on the receiving end of two traumatic experiences - I had first-hand experience.

I chose this format because I wanted you to understand where my beliefs and experiences have arisen from. Starting from my early years and my understanding of those formative experiences - through adversity, pain, discomfort and imbalance - pushing me right to the edge of understanding more about me - my mind, body, soul connection - then into *'freedom',* coming out the other side with a new profound perspective.

Each chapter starts with a quote, which I have personally written and is relevant to the chapter. The quotes can be used as affirmations if you so choose. Each chapter then takes you on a journey through my life, each finishing with a realisation section called *'A Way Will Be Found'.* Here is where I create a deeper understanding of how we can deal with adversity, feelings, beliefs and emotions, which we can then apply to our lives. Deep-seated beliefs can block your flow and communication. Understanding our thoughts, feelings and responses to circumstances in our lives can affect the outcome in reality. When we place our focus in the right direction and look at our challenges from a place of development and empowerment, we can shift from that place of adversity to true enlightenment.

The *'fear'* and isolation, which was once part of my life, now seems a distant memory. I hope to provide *'trust, faith and belief'* that **'a way will be found'** - that we can learn and navigate through any adversity, if we so choose, changing it to a positive outlook and experience. When we practise gratitude, kindness, self-respect and respect for others, having that *'trust, faith and belief'*, and being open to connect to other possibilities, it unlocks doors for us.

Working with my mind certainly was the making of me. It freed me to move forward in the right mindset, allowing me to create a healing within my mind and body. I had to get it down on paper, to share with you. This is why my book exists. It is my purpose and hope to ignite the spark of *'energy'* within you, to awaken those questions about life. If I can help just one person change their life for the better, then I have done my job. I thank you for taking the time to read this book. I hope when you reach the end you feel uplifted, fearless and feel connected to your new-found *'energy'* and guidance! I hope that my journey inspires you to create change and empowers you to connect into a powerful life - *'**from fear to freedom!**'*

Author's Note

This book is mainly about my life and the knowledge I have learnt from the adversity I have experienced.

Parts of my story have been omitted to protect the privacy of family and friends. This in no way affects the essence of my story and the journey I was encountering.

I am not a professional book writer, but I have done my best at this moment in time to ensure accuracy of detail in the pages that follow. Everyone mentioned in this memoir has given me permission to use their part in the story - which has been relevant in bringing this book to fruition.

Michelle Townsend

Part I
Journey Through Dis-ease

Michelle Townsend

Chapter 1

Inner Child Programs...

'When we experience discomfort deep within us, it's our
'inner child' calling ...

Transform this pain, use it as guidance - teaching us
where to shift our focus to what
we are wanting.'

~ Michelle Townsend

A s a child, I grew up in Dudley, West Midlands - a place called the 'Black Country'. So called because during the Industrial Revolution it became one of Britain's most industrialised areas. Coal mines, iron foundries and steel mills were producing a very high level of pollution in the area. Hence the skies were full of smoke from these factories and the term 'The Black Country' arose. 'Black Country born and bred' as we are proud to say. People are proud of the blood, sweat and hard work that runs through their ancestral family trees. My ancestors worked as brass founders, French polishers and coal miners. Proud of their heritage. The Black Country accent is distinctive, prominent and frequently subjected to teasing. We are proud of our heritage and even have our own Black Country Alphabet. How amazing is that?

My parents were quite young when I was born in 1970. Mom was 22 and Dad 21. They were married 11 months before I was born. Initially, we lived with my nan, then moved to a block of flats on the 17th floor. I can remember certain memories of Eve Hill Flats. One thing I don't remember, is being stuck in the lift with my mom. Mom reassures me that she didn't panic in that moment, unlike when I was about 6 weeks old when I sneezed and blood started coming down my nose. We were at my paternal grandparents and everyone went into panic mode. This was because my dad and uncle's older sister Patricia at 6 weeks old sneezed and burst a blood vessel, later passing away. It must have been awful for my nan and grandad losing their first born. Thankfully I was ok. When I was about 2 years old, we moved to a semi-detached house. This remained my family home until I got married in September 1993.

My parents never really ventured far. They were very much home birds, especially my mom. She was always happy when she was at home in her own space. We never really travelled far, apart from our holidays to Weston-Super-Mare, where my nan had a large static caravan. It was my second home and I absolutely loved it! Nan had been lucky enough to win the football pools back in the early 70s and had invested in the caravan. During our holidays there, Dad would sort out any maintenance needs for her. Nan rented it out most of the time, so we had to book our holiday dates in. The caravan was round the bay from Weston - a place called Sand Bay, Kewstoke. I had many happy times there, especially visiting the Shell Shop on the toll road. I used to buy shells and all things related to the sea from there.

My dad worked as a plater/welder at Round Oak Steel Works - not far from home, which was ideal for him. He loved that place. One of my earliest memories was going with Dad one Christmas morning to feed the work's cat - 'Sugarfoot'. Nicknamed 'Sugarfoot' because she had put her foot into

Dad's cup of tea with two sugars. It was a massive place. I can remember clearly seeing all the furnaces and rolling mills for the steel. I imagined it was a fascinating place to work. Dad was a very practical man. Everything he measured had to be to the nearest millimetre! As a plater/welder, it had to be! I enjoyed spending many hours with my dad as a youngster. He would show me how to measure and make things, explaining how things worked; especially showing me how to service my first car, my tango orange Mini Clubman 'T' reg. Changing the oil, cleaning the spark plugs, checking brakes, the list goes on. I couldn't do it now, but I knew a lot about engines back then! I found it fascinating.

When Dad was just 5 years old, he had a very serious accident and nearly lost his life. He had a house brick thrown at him, which hit the top of his head. As you can imagine, the implications of this were worrying for my grandparents. Dad's head was cut open and his skull cracked. He still has the scar and dent on the top of his head to this day. Thankfully, he survived after a long stint in hospital. I dread to think about how my grandparents responded to this situation; the fear of losing their 5-year-old son. It is possible that my grandparents wanted to protect my dad in the following months and years, possibly stopping him going to certain places; especially after losing their first child so young. Sadly, Dad had another serious accident at the age of 16. Whilst training to become a plumber, the rung on a wooden ladder snapped, he lost his footing and fell backwards landing on an upside-down wheelbarrow and broke his back. His bottom three vertebrae were broken, and he spent 12 months in plaster. This accident left him with constant back pain for the rest of his life. My nan and grandad certainly had their worries as parents. Imagine the 'energy' around all of that!

My maternal nan was very outgoing - taking Mom out and on holidays when she was younger, so where had my mom picked up this 'not going out' scenario from? Mom has always had a nervous disposition, but in times of trauma and emergency, her strength shone through. She always dealt with situations positively and practically. She was amazing! Her hidden strength was to help us more than we could ever realise in the coming years. I always remember Mom being around when I was younger. She was a stay-at-home mom. She had part time jobs working at a place called the BSR (Birmingham Sound Producers) as a power press operator, making record base plates in Stourbridge. She also worked at a place called Greenaways, tailoring trousers and later worked as a cleaner. Mom had a traumatic childhood dealing with illness. Maybe this was why she was nervous. She never really realised her own true strength, not drawing from the adversity that she had experienced. At an early age, Mom experienced Rheumatic Fever, losing her ability to walk. Initially, doctors were concerned it was polio. Every time nan and grandad tried to move her, she screamed out in agony. At the age of 5, she had to learn to walk again, causing her to miss the first couple of years at school. But before all this, Mom remembers being out on a coach trip which went under a low dark bridge - the sudden darkness caused severe shock for my mom and created an instant change within her. Rheumatic Fever later appeared. Could the shock have triggered the illness?

Known as 'Super Nan', my maternal nan lived until she was 99 years of age! We were so hoping that she would reach the grand old age of 100, but sadly it wasn't to be. All her grandchildren and great-grandchildren loved calling her 'Super-Nan'; it was like she was some superhero! She kept our family together. She was one of these 'grey pound' generations, travelling off to Spain - Benidorm and the like, in her retirement, five or six times a year. Nan really did know how to enjoy herself. I really do think that's why she lived to the grand age that she did, because of having a true zest for life, a purpose. Right up until she passed, she painted her nails to match her outfits. Scarfs, skirts, blouses, shoes and handbags would all match; they had to, otherwise she wouldn't wear them! I'm very much like my nan in that respect; everything must match perfectly. Maybe it's because we shared the same birthday. It's obvious where I've got that ancestral programming from! Which of course I'm very happy to keep!

As a child, I lacked confidence. Looking back on my experiences and what I understand now, I can see the pattern clearly. I spot it straight away, but with new-found knowledge, it is now easier to change. One pattern which stands out more than any other is 'communication', especially with regard to the EHS I experienced. As I got older, I used to be quite shy, or so it seemed to be at the time. I used to back away from things and not put myself forward; yet I always remember my mom saying to me ... *'Oh, you used to say hello to everyone, waving your hand to passers-by when you were in your pushchair. You loved talking to people.'* So, what changed there?

At the age of 5, I experienced a rather nasty accident in my back garden. It could have been life changing for me. I was playing in the dirt, digging, trying to copy my mom, who loved her garden (so my dad informs me). There was a small garden wall just in front of me. My lovely, very large, Pyrenean Mountain Dog called Snowy was also playing and running round the garden. I remember it being a lovely summer's day. I enjoyed the garden. Suddenly, as I was focused on digging the dirt, Snowy ran up the garden path, past me and knocked me forward at full force. Within a split second, I found my mom and dad running out to me, shouting their concern. Snowy had pushed me and my head had hit the corner of the wall. I hit the wall just above my left eye just below my eyebrow. Blood was gushing out and the next thing I can remember is being scrambled into the car, my mom holding me, with tea towels trying to cover the blood and stop the large cut bleeding. You can imagine as a parent what your thoughts would have been ... *'She's lost her eye! She could be blind!'* It must have been awful for my parents. At this time, the nearest hospital was in Birmingham. Mom kept telling me to stay awake during the long journey. I was starting to lose consciousness. I remember very clearly the nurse that took me under her wing when we arrived - the procedure of being stitched back together and the very large white handkerchief I was given afterwards. I can see myself lying on the stretcher type bed with the curtains around me now. The traumatic experience is imprinted on my brain as clear as if it was happening now. I still have the large scar just under my left eyebrow as a mascot to this day. Funny thing is, I don't remember the pain.

As I got older and more independent, I started to realise that there were other things to life. Up until then, it had been my holidays to Weston-Super-Mare and my music. Like I say, we never ventured far. I literally threw myself into my music. I know I sound very naïve here; I was, but suddenly I became aware that there were other things that people do in life. It started to open doors for me. But first, I had a lot to learn about fitting in, and I would learn this the hard way!

A Way Will Be Found

I had many moments where I felt lost as a child. I remember asking questions of myself such as ... *'Why am I here? What is this life all about?'* I'd look at the palm of my hands thinking ... *'How can this be real? How can I be real?'* Feeling baffled. This is amazing! Looking back, I was fascinated by life and reality.

As a youngster, I didn't have a deep understanding of how the mind worked, none of us do, unless we are taught it. As children we just flow through life without realising, absorbing the information around us, soaking it all up like a sponge. As children we are free to give our gifts of inspiration to the world. Living in the 'now' moment. It is such a beautiful thing to be inspired and show inspiration that just flows naturally from us. Most children do this - teaching adults what they have forgotten.

What if we are picking up responses from our parents that could be detrimental to us? Not intentionally of course. Most parents want the very best for their children. What if our parents have programming that they have never dealt with themselves? Programming that they picked up from their elders. Some people aren't even aware of their programming.

From the third trimester in our mother's womb through to age 7, we are building our personality traits from our experiences; watching and learning from people around us, how they respond, how things are dealt with. We learn how to respond; it is programmed into us and can be difficult to change. It's what shapes us as adults. I often wondered if people ask themselves ... *'Am I really my true self? Am I running other people's programs, copying them? What if I were to find the true self that is really me, and not that person that everyone else has had a dip into programming? What if I had a reset button?'* Asking these questions highlighted personality traits which weren't actually me! Realising that the old programming was running, seeing it from a new perspective, as an adult, meant that I could then start to address and change it for the better - through the power of thought. That's where powerful change can happen - where life can be changed for the better!

Ever heard the saying ... *'Give me a child until he is 7 and I will show you the man'?*[1] The words of Aristotle the Greek philosopher. Birth to age 7 is the most crucial time for development and learning, and obviously programming in a child. As a parent with young babies, ask the question ... *'What would I like my child to become?'* Watch what you are allowing into their awareness. How do you talk to them? Do you inspire them, or do you knock them down? Even though most of our programming goes on at this early age, I still believe our true *'inner child'* exists; the part that exists before any programming. Our natural instincts develop from previous generations, evolution and even past lives.

When anyone experiences something traumatic, including the associated strong feelings and emotions, it leaves impressions on them that run very deep. It can be life changing, creating beliefs, responses and perceptions in one foul swoop! There is a part of our mind that wants to protect us - our subconscious. Traumatic life situations happen to us. How people respond during and after the trauma can create responses and beliefs that carry through the rest of our lives. The question is are these responses really needed? Are they beneficial to us? Do they create blockages that can stifle our future choices as an adult?

My dad, as a youngster, would have thought nothing about his parents' responses, believing it to be normal life. This is how we are. However, he would have picked up the *'protection energy'* that he was being engulfed in. This, in turn, could have caused his responses as an adult to be concerned about where he went and what he did. I may be completely wrong here, but there's a possibility that this program still subconsciously runs in my dad even now, without him realising. My grandparents wouldn't even have thought they were doing anything wrong; in fact, they weren't. However, from their responses, you can certainly see what it could create further down the line. All done through love, with no intention of creating adverse responses. It's interesting when you are made aware of perception, isn't it? We can't go down the road of the blame game here. Responses appear for a reason. We do our best in any situation. Was my mom's subconscious finding a way to protect her from the outside world? All illness is energetic, whether we believe it to be or not. Illness can be created from an experience, response, or feeling - which does not necessarily have to be traumatic either. Louise Hay's book 'You Can Heal

Your Life'[2] gives a full description of this. If the response is not dealt with emotionally, it can manifest physically. The mind puts things in place to protect us from the original experience, it can create any response. It thinks it is doing its best for you.

As I have got older, I have become aware that because my parents weren't very adventurous, maybe I energetically picked up those traits in my childhood. The *'energy'* my parents would have been emitting about not venturing out to places and the feelings related to that, surely, I would have sensed? Now I'm not in any way saying what my parents chose to do was wrong. There is no right or wrong. What they did was comfortable and right for them. However, I would have been taught those responses as a child - not being too adventurous or feeling confident about going out for meals etc; not venturing to new places. This doesn't have to be spoken words, we just naturally pick up the **'energy'**.

Reality is what we see from our own perspective, beliefs and expectations. Everyone has a different view on what's in front of them; we all respond very differently. Our responses to positive or difficult situations have been dictated, prescribed and reinforced to us by how our peers and parents respond. Their response comes from a culture of expectation. We learn from these role models by watching, listening and copying. It's no different to learning a musical instrument really, and you can be taught that correctly or incorrectly. We all have our own way, there's no right or wrong way to do things. We find our own way in the end.

Using the negative as guidance allows a refocus. Bringing forward a learning, allowing a step forward in our new powerful potential *'energy'* where we can transform *'fear',* anger, frustration and sadness - using those feelings to redirect and allow powerful change. This can benefit us if we take on the perspective of addressing the negative in a productive way. It's just a matter of looking at life from a different perspective, not believing everything we are told. We do have our own 'inner guidance' and usually it is right for us. We are all unique and different. Learn to question thoughts!

What do I mean by this 'inner guidance'? Sometimes called our 'inner child'. Simply, it's our 'true self'. We all have gut feelings. Feelings that make us feel excited, happy, content, comfortable, safe, secure, loved, reassured ... the list goes on. There are also gut feelings of apprehension, unhappiness, insecurity, uncomfortableness, things that don't sit right with us, making us feel unloved, unsafe, unsure. No matter who we are when we are born, we hold our own true 'inner guidance' within us, and our feelings are our indicators. Feelings come from the subconscious, it's the emotional part of our mind. We can use our feelings to help guide and direct what's right and wrong for us. We have our own soul, irrelevant to our parents. The reset button comes from that natural soul guidance. It is there if you choose to connect with it and bring awareness to it. We have all experienced decisions where we didn't follow our gut instinct and learned a harsh lesson from it. 'I should have followed my gut instinct' is usually our comment.

Programming is what has shaped us as adults today, but we do have a deeper choice, a personal choice. We are only connected to our past by the thoughts and beliefs we hold. I chose to check in with my gut feelings. Really questioned how I felt at a particular moment in time. 'How did I normally respond?' Or should I say ... 'How had I been 'taught to respond? Was it the right response for me?' It was amazing what came forward.

Go with what comes from deep within you. Choose what feels right in any moment. You will then usually make the right choice and response for YOU, from your 'true self'. Reparent your 'inner child'. Teach your young ones that and empower them!

References:

[1] Aristotle. (350 BCE). *Give me a child until he is 7 and I'll show you the man.* In R. McKeon (Ed.), The Basic Works of Aristotle (pp. 123-124). Random House.

[2] Hay, L. (1984). *You Can Heal Your Life.* Hay House.

Michelle Townsend

Chapter 2

Fitting In

'Send out that big, wonderful bubble of energy that is YOU ...
Remember you are AMAZING!
Be proud of it!'

~ Michelle Townsend

It was my first day attending infants school and I wanted to escape! I remember being in that classroom. Within the first few days I decided to walk out! I wanted to go home. I didn't want to be there. The teacher shouted and asked where I was going? I know this is probably what most young children feel as they start school at the age of 5. It's all very daunting for us as little ones, but nevertheless I wanted to go home.

I can't remember a great deal from infants school, I just remember wanting to leave, feeling lost, being at home seemed better. I'm not saying it was totally awful. It wasn't. I had many happy times; it was just that feeling of being lost that seemed to run in the background, ticking away subtlety. Little did I realise that in the end, infants and juniors were to be the best part of my school days.

It's funny what we remember. There are always memories that are linked with strong emotion - good and bad. The subconscious part of our mind locks these memories away for keeping, sometimes raising their 'ugly head' when you least expect it! Although infants school is far from my memory vault, I do remember a few things that stuck in my mind. Especially when I was hit by the playground bell. There were lots of children in the corridor, all crammed together in a small area. I think it was a very rainy day and I was standing right by the teacher, who had got the old traditional bronze bell for playtime. Next thing I knew...whallop! Right on the top of my head. It's a wonder it didn't knock me out! Probably knocked some sense into me more like! The teacher apologised and asked if I was ok, rubbed the top of my head better, then we just carried on and went into our classrooms. The response wouldn't be like that nowadays; accident book, parents being told etc. It was me that told my mom. Nothing was said to her from the school back then. I swear that's why I have a slight dent on the top of my head! I was concerned about that dent when I had to have all my hair shaved off during my chemotherapy treatment, but it wasn't all that big of a bronze bell impression on my head after all!

At junior school, I can recall my friend, Julie, telling me John Lennon had died. I can still remember where we were standing in the cloakroom corridor area, waiting to go into our classroom.

"Who?" I said.

I hadn't a clue who John Lennon was! We would have been about 10 at the time. Once Julie informed me he was one of The Beatles, I realised straight away. I've always been rubbish at remembering names; good at numbers, but not names. My pupils continue to laugh at me even now when I can't remember the composer names whilst I'm teaching.

I always found myself feeling tense a great deal of the time at school - I just couldn't relax in that environment. I just had this stressful uncomfortable feeling going on. I remember sitting at the dinner table in the school dining room. We were all sitting around a large round table. It was almost a feeling of being embarrassed to eat in front of people; it would just come over me. Silly really. I'd taken a 'Pot Noodle' and a flask of hot water. I literally felt really embarrassed whilst I was preparing it, but why? Friends sitting round the table did ask if I was ok, so I obviously showed some form of being uncomfortable. I was always conscious of people looking at me, watching me, wondering what they were thinking. I still get this feeling now occasionally. Certain beliefs never seem to leave you; they are deep seated personality traits that are hard to shift.

Having something stolen from you for the first time leaves deep seated memories, because it creates that strong emotional feeling of being threatened indirectly. It is a feeling of disappointment with the person concerned. You almost feel sad for them, that they have had to resort to this; it sticks with you. As well as sympathy, you feel angry and upset. I remember the first time this happened to me. It was a keyring with a world on it, a small metal ball on a chain. I had shown it to my friends who were sitting around the table. The keyring was attached to my school bag. I left the classroom to go to the toilet, only to return to find the keyring gone! No one knew anything. I questioned everyone at the table. Deep down, my gut instinct told me who had taken it. It was obvious to me ... but could I have been wrong? That person had shown specific interest in the keyring and had been messing around with it, teasing me, taking it off my bag and off me. I can even remember the person's name and what they looked like. I never saw it again! Children can be horrible! This really upset me deeply, that a so-called friend who was sitting at my table, wasn't trustworthy. That triggered and created responses in me to become more protective of my things from then on. Why does someone do that? I just didn't get it! I understand now that people only respond from their needs and wants. Maybe this child felt deprived in some way - or was jealous. Who knows? Did it make them feel better?

At the age of 8 years and 4 months, I became a sister. This helped with how I was feeling at school. I had a new focus. On the day my sister was born, Dad took me to have my ears pierced. I had been pestering Mom and Dad for ages, asking if I could have them done. They were hesitant - but, what a lovely surprise to be taken to the jewellers to get them done that day. It was so exciting! I remember the lady marking where the piercing was going to go; we agreed, then using a piercing gun I had my ears pierced. It didn't hurt at all. I wanted to look after my new piercings myself; after all, I was a 'new big sister' now. But 6 weeks later, when Mom took them out to try new earrings, I fainted flat out on the kitchen floor. It made me feel weird as she took them out. I hadn't been cleaning them with surgical spirit properly. That was a lesson learned! All was resolved in the end. Being an older sister, I took on board a mother nurturing aspect. I just wanted to love and look after my new baby sister. It was almost like I was playing Mom. I enjoyed every moment with my sister as she grew from a baby to a toddler. We had many happy times, never arguing as some sisters do. Just enjoying being sisters together.

After infants and junior school, my best friend, Julie, decided she was going to attend the senior school which her brothers had. I was gutted! I really would have loved to have started senior school together. I felt I had no friend to start the next leg of the school journey with. I know that's not true as I had many wonderful friends, but I was always very quiet. I would always avoid saying what I thought and not speak up. Keeping myself to myself. Could that come from being pulled up about not answering back to my elders? It was just my thoughts about something which I was voicing, but always told not to answer back. I believe it created a habit for not speaking up or having the confidence to speak up. That's how I saw it and how

I picked it up. I always felt the odd one out, to be honest. I hated it! The feelings I was experiencing confused me, baffled me. Why did I find it all so hard? Does everyone else feel the same?

It was a long walk to senior school, so I had to set out a good 40 minutes before to get there on time. I walked to school with various friends from the cul-de-sac where we lived. There were lots of children my age in our street. The 40-minute walk home allowed me time to buy a king size Mars bar to chobble on. I loved that treat! We had many great times 'playing out' over the years. My one friend had a brilliant willow tree in her garden. It was massive! We used to climb it most weeks, incredibly high up too. The gardens looked over to the Fens Nature Reserve. From some gardens, there was access through to the Fens Pool. One afternoon, whilst climbing a tree over the Fens by the willow tree, I suddenly slipped and fell, landing in a mass of tall nettles below. My legs, hands and side of my body were in agony from the number of stings. Not wise falling out of trees! I tended to like being upside-down doing gymnastics! I also had a habit of coming off my bike. Looking round to see where your friend is as you are literally bombing at speed down the road, to then realise as you turn back and look in front of you, there is a parked car. You hit the back of the car, go 'arse over tip' and land on your face! Yup, I did that! Lovely big scab for weeks all on the one side of my face, as you do! We had loads of fun in our street! My mom used to call me a *"Chap my wench".* In other words, a girl who was very boyish. A Black Country term there for you! Dad bought a brand-new trials motorbike in 1983. I remember it was an 'A' registration. Thankfully I didn't have a habit of falling off that! I used to love being a passenger on the back of Dad's motorbike. I even had my own helmet.

I found school tiring, picking up the *'energy'* around me. I was an empath. I would always listen to what people were going through, putting myself in their shoes, trying to understand their feelings. It made me feel uncomfortable. I understand it fully now. I wasn't allowing myself to be me, not speaking up, not standing up for myself. I just wanted to fit in, putting others first. There were situations like friends asking to look through my bag, obviously I would oblige, I'd do anything to feel I fitted in, thinking they would like me more. A real cheek, to ask to look through someone's bag, their personal belongings; especially when you had things in your bag like sanitary towels hiding at the bottom. I was just a young girl, embarrassed enough already, without someone pulling my belongings out of my bag; in front of a class full of teenagers. But there you go, it happened. I don't hold it against them. Now I understand that's what young mischievous teenagers do. I tended not to tease though, I always respected people's feelings and boundaries around me. Was it because I was always quiet and an easy target? Was it how I was brought up? I never wanted to upset anyone and just wanted to get on with everyone. I've never liked animosity; I don't like negative *'energy'*. I just couldn't understand how people could be like this. I realise now it was the *'energy'*. We all give off *'energy'*, we are all electromagnetic beings; it's how we resonate with each other. That's why we get on with some people and not others. There's nothing wrong with that. The *'energy'* I was emitting myself was through *'fear'*; I was focused on *'fear'* - fear of what was going to happen next? Thus, reality gave me something to fear, it matched the frequency, it became my reality. It was where I was focused. Where to sit and who with? I literally felt like a lost soul. All I could think about was that my best friend wasn't with me. My stomach would churn, concerning myself of where I would be in each class. I hated senior school for the first three years.

For a while, I arrived at school early to prepare coffee for the headmistress. I did this along with another girl. I don't remember how we got asked to do this, but we used to sort coffee out for the percolator. It made us feel quite special helping the headmistress, but it eventually fizzled out after a couple of years.

There were some lovely people at school, and I had some amazing friends, but there were also some I didn't quite connect with. In life, there are always people we don't hit it off with or don't resonate with. I don't hold that against anyone, I understand the rules of life and I wish them well. I just wish I had more understanding of this at that early age. I used to think it was me. It really is just part of life that we get on with certain people better than others. If we were all the same, it would be a pretty boring world, wouldn't it? Because of all this, I didn't want to stay at school during the lunch hour. I would venture off to my nan's. Mondays, Wednesdays and Fridays were spent with my paternal grandmother, then Tuesdays and Thursdays with my maternal grandmother. This allowed me to spend more time with them over the years; I'm so glad I did. It was great having home-cooked egg and chips for lunch! Neither lived far from school, so a quick walk and I was there in no time.

For as long as I can remember, my nickname was 'Rubber Lips!' Yes, I do have more voluptuous lips which I happen to be very proud of now! Most women pay out ridiculous amounts of money to get lips like mine! I hated that part of me, how I looked. Again, I was embarrassed. I would feel hurt, upset, find it difficult to let go, take it personally. I would be teased left, right and centre about my lips. I also had a gap in my teeth, but no one seemed to tease me about that, thankfully. That gap eventually closed. When Madonna became famous, back in the 80s, I used to look at her and think … *'That's like my teeth, Madonna has a gap in hers too,'* … so that made it alright. Mine was starting to close at this point, but it was something that I'd also been very conscious of for many years.

The uneasiness continued at school. Bullying is horrible! Apparently, I'd been a 'grass' and had 'grassed' someone up! I still don't know to this day what I was supposed to have grassed about or who it was, but it went on for ages, years in fact. The stairs in school used to wind round, covering the four floors. There were two staircases. At the top of the landing, was a small square area. This is where I was nearly pushed over the edge of the banister, deliberately! I'd spend weekends curled up on the settee at home, feeling low, worrying about going to school on a Monday morning again.

After a couple of years, Julie was not settling in her new school. She was unhappy. Things were soon put in place for her to move school to continue her education. It was great to have her on the journey through our final years at senior school. I eventually started to feel I had settled down. I started to enjoy school. However, within a blink of an eye, it was time to leave. Maybe that was the reason I settled down; I don't know? Maybe because I was coming to the end of my time at school. Perhaps there was a sense of relief deep within me, but I never, truly relaxed there.

A Way Will Be Found

Not everyone gets on; it's true! I had great difficulty understanding this as a child. I just wanted to be friends with everyone, no bad vibes, or feelings. Creating a deep understanding that we are all different, with our own views and outlooks, can allow us to let go of any negativity we are faced with. When honouring that for each other, the flow through life is so much easier. We are all unique.

Empaths find this difficult to do. Empaths are oversensitive to people's emotions and responses, owning their 'energy'. These emotions and responses are not ours to own, that's just someone else's perspective. Everyone is brought up differently. We all develop different perspectives from our own experiences and what we have been taught from our peers and parents. If taught from an early age, we can learn from our experiences, navigating life better. This isn't on everyone's radar, but children certainly create misunderstandings from their experiences.

We do all require a sense of belonging. When someone confronts us, it can be hard to accept. We start to turn inwardly, lack confidence, back away, find it difficult to speak up - just like I did. That was all I could understand back then. Being an empath, it is much harder to deal with. With the realisation of 'not everyone gets on', I'm sure things would have been different for me. Teach children the simplicities of this. It's not difficult to understand; it may even seem silly, but it can be far reaching to a youngster's mind. Understanding creates empowerment within.

It is important to understand that 'a sense of belonging is important to both our mental and physical health'. It's one of our basic *'human needs'*. We all require certain things to survive, to live in this world, and these vary from person to person. When those human needs aren't met or are not being fully acknowledged, then certain responses, behaviour and experiences can occur. Maslow's Hierarchy of needs (1943)[1] represents such needs. These needs move from the most basic to the most advanced. *'Basic'* needs must first be met before anyone can move up to more advanced *'self-fulfilling needs'.*

Basic Needs

Psychological Needs – Breathing, Water, Food, Warmth, Rest, Reproduction.

Safety Needs – Security, Safety, Employment, Resources, Property, Health.

Psychological Needs

Love and Belonging Needs – Friendship, Intimate relationships, Family, Connection.

Esteem Needs – Self-esteem, Confidence, Respect, Recognition, Achievement, Accomplishment, Purpose, Freedom.

Self-fulfilment Needs

Self-actualization Needs – Achieving one's full potential, Creative activities, Exploration.

These needs appear to be the standard, simplistic basic things of life. But what if one of those needs is missing from your hierarchy? Ask yourself what creates motivation in me? What turns you on? What floats your boat? It's all to do with motivation. It also relates to purpose. If we haven't got purpose in our lives, there's no point; that's when we feel lost, closed-down, unimportant.

This leads me to an interesting long-term experiment which continues to this day. The *'Harvard Experiment of Adult Development'*[2] (Waldinger, 1938) included a total of 724 men from all types of backgrounds and environments. The experiment was researching what made people live longer and is now expanding to their children. Every two years, the men are questioned, interviewed, have medical aspects checked and receive a scan on their brains. The men are questioned about their relationships.

Could relationships keep us happier and healthier? The experiment established that social connections are good for us. Loneliness kills. People who are more isolated from others, find that they are less happy, they decline quicker. People who communicate with others, attend social events, venture out more, have better relationships and quality of life. It is the quality of our relationships that is important to us. Good relationships protect our brains and help us live longer. My nan was a perfect example of this experiment, living to the grand old age of 99. She certainly proved this to be true! The good life is built with good relationships.

'There isn't time, so brief is life, for bickerings, apologies, heartburnings, callings to account. There is only time for loving, and but an instance so to speak, for that.'[3]

~ Mark Twain

So, what did I gain from all these feelings? These realisations? What was the teaching in all of this? Well, it certainly took its time! Acknowledging how we feel in any moment is highlighting what's right or wrong for us. Remember our 'gut instinct'? We need to respect each other's differences, but in the first instance have the deeper understanding that we are all unique. We are all allowed to be ourselves. Avoid the arguments, no one is right or wrong, we are allowed our own point of view even if others don't agree. It's how we learn as part of this amazing world. Share our differences, so we can learn and look at things in different ways. It's important to be true to ourselves, not just for ourselves, but for others. Something I learned the hard way.

References:

[1] Maslow, A. H. (1943). *A theory of human motivation. Psychological Review,* Vol 50 No 4 370-396.

[2] Waldinger, R. (1938, p. 123). *The Harvard Experiment of Adult Development.* Harvard University.

[3] Twain, M., & Twichell, J. H. (2017). *The Letters of Mark Twain and Joseph Hopkins Twichell.* University of Georgia Press.

Michelle Townsend

Chapter 3

Music was My First Love

*'When the time is right, things fall into place.
Let go of the disappointment, it's there for a reason ... to grow!'*

*'The gentle tones of music connect us to the flow of life ... just
like notes flow melodically ... allow connection to harmony
within you.'*

~ Michelle Townsend

*'Music was my first love, and it will be my last. Music of the
future, and music of the past. To live without my music, would
be impossible to do. For in this world of troubles, my music pulls
me through.'*[1]

~ John Miles

For as long as I can remember, I've always had a keen interest in music. From around the age of 7, Dad showed me how to play electronic organ, teaching me to play by ear at first. We had an old 'Thomas' organ. Playing in a band for a while, Dad was a keen guitarist, but also had an interest in keyboards. I remember the very first song he taught me - 'Spanish Eyes'[2] - adding an introduction which involved a musical technique I now know of as playing in thirds. It was great! Dad always added his own extra riffs to his playing, experimenting and improvising, which I thought was amazing as a youngster. Organs were all the rage back in the 1970s. Many bands owned 'Hammond' organs, especially rock bands; still using these to this day. 'Hammond' organs are particularly known for their famous tremolo and 'Leslie' speaker effects. They have a brilliant, distinct sound.

I continued to show a real interest in playing electronic organ and by the age of 12, had started lessons, learning music properly. I loved it. Within 12 months of starting, I was entered for the 'Grade 2' practical examination with 'Southern Music Training Centre', gaining a merit, which I was ecstatic about! 'Southern Music Training Centre' had been created especially for electronic organ exams.

I continued to work through my practical exams, being invited to perform in concerts and presentations via the music school. It was here I met my husband-to-be. I first remember seeing Karl when I was around 12/13 years old. We were being presented with our certificates from our recent music exams. Little did I realise that we would be married ten years later!

The concerts we both took part in were at our local Town and Civic Halls. It was a big thing, very nerve racking but an amazing feeling. It was in one of these concerts that Karl and my teacher dressed up to do Offenbach's 'Can-Can'[3]. I was performing a duet with my teacher of the 'Hooked on Classics'[4] medley. They both came on stage with wigs on. My word! Did we have fun in those concerts! Such a laugh! Again, at this point, I never thought I would be married to Karl; we just enjoyed the musical aspect of being part of a lovely music centre.

From starting my lessons, the desire to become a music teacher was planted in my mind. I enjoyed the lessons and music so much. Along with the amazing concerts, I started to play in local pubs in our area. At 15, I was playing on a Thursday night in a pub opposite Russells Hall Hospital. Our electronic organ was transported there with the help of my dad's friend. *'Free and easy with Michelle'* the poster said - not a phrase you would use nowadays as it would probably be interpreted in quite a different way! I still have that poster. I then became resident organist at a pub called 'The Wagon and Horses' in Cradley Heath for a while. I used to look forward to my Sunday evenings entertaining the locals. It was around this time that I invested in a new instrument which was more portable, allowing me to transport it to gigs easier. The Technics EX30L was just the ticket; it was much smaller. I also bought two Technics speaker amps SY-T15s; they were perfect and had a great sound. During my gigging days, I became known as the 'Sandy Shaw' of organ players, playing with no shoes - bare foot. That all started at a concert at the Station Hotel, Dudley, when a famous organist commented on my bare feet. I'd pinched a piece of music he was going to perform that evening, Billy Joel's 'Root Beer Rag'[5]. He kindly let me perform it. The comments about my feet then followed me everywhere. I also started a Saturday job, teaching beginners, along with my current teacher. I loved it! Teaching beginners was the start of my journey to what eventually led to the establishing of my music business of 37 years! Eventually, I was left running the music school where I had started, branching out on my own. I registered as self-employed in July 1987 at just 17 years old and never looked back.

Music played a key part in my life. At junior school, we had a lovely teacher, Mrs Burrows. My best friend Julie and I started to learn the recorder. Once again, I took part in everything I could to do with music. Julie and I became part of the recorder group. We also became a big part of the shows our school organised; it was just great! Mrs Burrows was such a lovely music teacher; however, she did put our noses out of joint once. Both Julie and I wanted to be part of the cast Christmas production.

Mrs Burrows made it quite clear ... *"No! You are part of my band and I need you both on recorder, so you can't go for a part in the production!"*

We were gutted, but we still loved that we were a big part of it all. It's funny when you look back at your childhood. We were always singing and dancing too, especially when Bucks Fizz won the 1981 Eurovision with 'Making Your Mind Up.'[6] We enjoyed singing and dancing. I still have a tape recording of us singing 'Give It Up'[7] by KC and The Sunshine Band somewhere. Such happy memories. We were so engrossed in music that we applied to go on 'Peter Craig's Beacon Radio Show'. Julie loved Peter Craig. We finally won a place on the show and were so excited. Dad took us to the studios in Tettenhall, Wolverhampton. What an amazing experience.

Music was the theme and focus throughout my school days; it was my mainstay; it kept me sane. Once Julie was back at senior school with me, we would get together - I would play and Julie would sing. We were always singing at my house too - must have driven my mom mad! When it came to our final school exams, I decided to use my 'Grade 7' organ pieces for my performance. I had just taken my 'Grade 7' exam, so they were polished pieces ready to go. I had quite a repertoire to choose from at this time. Pieces such as 'Hello'[8], 'Up Where We Belong'[9], 'Root Beer Rag', 'Organ Hoedown'[10] - the list goes on. I played various genres: modern, classical, jazz, plus many pieces arranged for electronic organ specifically; but it was right to choose my 'Grade 7' pieces of which 'Moonglow'[11] was one. Such a beautiful piece with lovely flowing melodic jazz passages. It was a cracker! Around May 1986, a lady examiner arrived at my house to examine me for school. It was difficult to move the organ, so all was arranged for a special visit. I remember her being about 7 months pregnant. I passed with flying colours!

It was at this time in my life where I took a deep interest in ghosts, hauntings, spirits and the occult. I was fascinated by supernatural things in life, much to my mom's dismay! I have no idea what made me aware of these things, but I just knew there was something else more than this reality. I would talk to my friends about it whilst out in the street and at school. Watching a Ouija board experience certainly opened my eyes. Thankfully I was only an observer at that séance. I even used the book 'The Amityville Horror'[12] (Anson, 1977) as part of my reading and presentation for my elocution lessons and exam at college. At one point I felt a deep connection being made by my paternal grandmother who had passed away in hospital. Music created the connection as she passed over. The experience was phenomenal! I feel this was the very start of my connection to understanding the deeper aspect of the mind and higher *'energy'* realm - that there was something more out there.

My choices after leaving school disappointed me. After looking at continuing with my music studies, I was told that electronic organ wasn't an accepted instrument to continue into further education, *'WHAT?'* Gutted was an understatement. It's different nowadays; electronic instruments can get you into university. It made sense why the 'Southern Music Training Centre' had been created. Back then, electronic organs weren't classed as recognised instruments. They were a phenomenal examination board for the instrument, certainly doing Karl and myself proud. I hadn't started piano at this time, so that wasn't an option either. If I was looking at college today to study music, there are so many choices and options, but it wasn't to be back in the mid-80s. I made the choice to do a secretarial course, including law. I looked at it as a backup for my music. I still desperately wanted a career in music, so I continued with my music privately. It was my only option at this time, but I was determined!

College didn't go that well. Whilst at home one Friday afternoon September 1986, there was a knock at the door.

Mom had gone to fetch my sister from school. It was my dad's workmate.

"Is your mom in?" ... he asked, as I opened the door.

"No, she's gone to fetch my sister," I replied. *"What's wrong?"*

"Your dad has been rushed to Sandwell Hospital, he collapsed at work, he's had a heart attack!"

To say I was shocked was an understatement!

"What do I do? I need to go and tell Mom."

At that, Dad's friend left for the hospital in a rush. He'd obviously done the job of coming to notify us in person. I then ran as fast as I could to school to tell my mom - mobile phones weren't around then. Whilst running I had thoughts about how my dad hadn't been himself the last month or so. He had been complaining about pains in his left arm and had been sweating a lot whilst decorating my bedroom, stopping to take a rest. Funny - as it was coincidental that the wallpaper he happened to be putting on my bedroom wall was white with red love hearts on it! We teased him and blamed the wallpaper! He was only 37. *'How could he have a heart attack at 37?'* I don't even remember running to the school - no idea how I got there! I told Mom, who was distraught. Things were then put in place for us to go to the hospital. It was my sister's birthday the following day. A party had been planned to take place at home. Mom was determined for this to go ahead, as it was the first big party she had organised for my sister. Dad was in a bad way. He'd had a massive heart attack which had damaged most of the lower part of his heart. The hospital visit brought the realisation of what had actually happened. In ICU, Dad was wired up to machines everywhere, which were bleeping. Drugs were keeping him alive and easing the pain. He looked ill. The emergency team had used a defibrillator on Dad as they were rushing him through the hospital doors. As we left that evening, doctors told my mom that the next 24/48 hours were crucial. It was possible he could have another heart attack. We left with the worry of what the weekend might bring. Mom got up early the next day and cleaned the house top to bottom - she couldn't sit still. All the worry was making her agitated but determined for the party to go ahead. I helped as much as I could, and we got through my sister's 8th birthday party; we kept our chins up. It was just a shame Dad wasn't there to share it with us! Dad survived his critical ordeal, spending the next several months recovering at home.

Through all this, I had to continue with college. My heart wasn't in it, but I did my best. Sadly, my attendance started to suffer after becoming ill with Glandular Fever, also known as Epstein Barr Virus. Not something else to deal with! My energy levels were rock bottom, and I would find myself falling asleep in lessons, to then be sent home. The Head of Faculty would ring home to see how I was and why I wasn't attending college. Between you and me, I was still managing to do some teaching work during the evenings. Music was my first love; that's where my heart was. I would do anything to continue that - anything! Mom and Dad suggested I looked at my options - continue college or turn completely to my music.

After just 12 months at college, I left. I'd had enough. I wasn't following my heart. I made the decision to become self-employed as a private music teacher. I was only teaching beginners at the time, but this developed later into teaching higher grades. I finally took my 'Grade 8', and after passing my driving test in December 1987 (first time too!) I left the music studios and became a private, mobile music teacher, visiting pupils privately for their lessons. Driving allowed me to travel, so I did. This was my life for a while. I loved my job. Seeing pupils develop their skills as players was just fabulous!

In 1988, it was decided to transform a room at Mom and Dad's, allowing me to do some teaching from home. Karl - now an electrical apprentice, offered to help with the alterations. By the end of January 1989, Karl and I had started dating attending many rock concerts. We were rockers at heart! I carried on teaching from my parents' house and continued mobile visits until July 1992, when Karl and I bought our own house. It took just a total of two weeks from viewing to holding the keys in our hands! During a trip to Florida in the September, 'Black Wednesday' happened and we thought we had lost our house, but everything settled by the time we returned. It was whilst on this trip, my fear of lifts appeared. We were on a deep-sea simulator ride when I suddenly became claustrophobic wanting to get off. The ride had already started. Telling myself it was just a simulator and closing my eyes seemed to help, but this triggered my fear of enclosed spaces and lifts from that point. Where had this arisen from?

Karl and I were engaged in December 1992. As soon as I could, I transferred all my teaching to our new home. Mom and Dad had put up with me long enough, which I was very grateful for, but it was time to move on. I moved into our new home when Karl and I were married in September 1993. Until then, I'd just stayed weekends. I liked it that way. On the morning of my wedding day, I watched the sun rise. It was such a wonderful day saying 'I do' at 2pm. Karl surprised me with a trip to Austria for our honeymoon - only finding out at our evening reception where we were going. It was a lovely surprise. Even our honeymoon was music based - visiting Mozart's birthplace in Salzburg.

Karl and I were happily married; life was going well. We had a lot of work to do on the house, but it was liveable. Karl completely rewired the house, and we worked through each room at a time. It was fun!

In the years that followed, I further developed my own standards and Continuing Professional Development (CPD), going on to complete my 'Teaching Diploma' in December

1996 with 'Guildhall School of Music and Drama'. My uncle would accompany me once a fortnight to Nuneaton, where I had lessons with a wonderful lady called Paule. She helped me tremendously and I will always be extremely grateful for that time and development. Paule was a teacher and examiner. I invested in a piano around the age of 20, taking piano exams, adding to my achievements. I would also sit for hours doing theory. I loved it! Even on days out when Karl was windsurfing, I'd sit in the car reading and writing music theory. Music was my life! Eventually, the electronic organ gradually faded out and electronic keyboard - a single keyboard instrument with what we call 'automatic play chord' facility became more popular. During the 90s keyboards took over. It was a great instrument, but I still loved organ and piano more. I've had some amazing Technics keyboards over the years. I now have the KN7000, the last one they made. Phenomenal orchestral sound; you are your own little orchestra. I still have the KN3000, which my son has with him in London. You were either a 'Technics' or 'Yamaha' lover. Technics all the way with me! Our Technics GA3 organ, which I took my teaching diploma on, still sits in our lounge. Now, piano is my main instrument along with music theory. I'm still going strong and very proud of my music school.

A Way Will Be Found

When we really want something, really crave a specific thing in any moment, we put forward the request of having it. We have a focus. That focus then starts to form. We start to see things falling into place in the reality around us. We give off the 'energy' of that focus. Continuing to feed that focus puts situations in place to allow your dream to come into fruition. You see, I knew what I wanted - I had that focus. It maybe didn't flow in the way I initially intended, but none the less I found 'a way'. I was determined. I found a way to continue my music. When we remember that there's no right or wrong way to achieve a goal; that there is only the right way for ourselves, other possibilities appear before us. Everyone's route will be a different experience. I'm not a university graduate. I didn't go to music college, but I found a way to allow music to flow in my life, choosing the private tuition route to get there! I'm still going! We never stop, we are always evolving!

Back then, I found music was my saviour. I would shut myself away, playing music to dampen the feelings deep within me that were frustrating me - not understanding certain parts of life, not understanding how people could be so different and treat us the way they did. I found comfort in my music. It was a clear focus and of course an achievement. It made me feel good.

We can navigate through life, even if we believe we can't. The road ahead may not be clear, but the drive to find our way takes over us, bringing in our intuition, being drawn into what feels good. Learn to connect with what feels good. You then have a much better chance of finding that 'inner child', that 'inner guidance path', that 'true self'. Almost certainly experiencing that 'fitting in' in the place that's right for you.

Richard Branson followed his heart and is a prime example of connecting into what feels good, bringing forward intuition and inspiration. Starting with a small business from his bedroom as a teenager, who would have thought that Branson would later own his own airline 'Virgin' and 'Necker Island' in the territory of the British Virgin Islands? Aren't we all flying by the seat of our pants each and every day anyway? It's part of the journey of life.

'If someone offers you an opportunity but you are not sure you can do it, say yes - then learn how to do it later!'[13]

~ Richard Branson

As human beings, we put things in place naturally to overcome other aspects of our life. We do this without realising it. Just like self-sabotage can take place, I believe self-saviour can too.

Back then, I experienced a tremendous amount of lack in confidence; but in the powerful words of John Miles's song 'Music', 'my music pulls me through'. There is always a way through if we look hard enough and keep our focus where we wish to be! Little did I realise that I would be keeping a strong focus and making decisions just like these in the future, which would save my life! Learning that my personality was indeed stronger than I thought, I realised that once I made a decision to move forward with specific choices, I maintained and stuck with my focus right to the end! It was time to connect and honour that within me! That's where my power resided!

References:

[1] Miles, J. (1976). *Music.* [Vinyl] London: Decca Records.

[2] Snyder, E., & Singleton, C. (1965). *Spanish Eyes.* [recorded by] 'Martino, A.' Capitol Records.

[3] Offenbach, J. (1858). *Can-can.* Orpheus in the Underworld. Operetta.

[4] Clark, L., & Royal Philharmonic Orchestra. (1981). *Hooked on Classics.* [K-tel]

[5] Joel, B. (1974). *Root Beer Rag.* Streetlife Serenade. Columbia Records.

[6] Hill, A., & Danter, J. (1981). *Making Your Mind Up.* [Recorded by] 'Bucks Fizz'. 1981 Eurovision. RCA.

[7] Casey, H.W., & Carter, D. (1981). *Give It Up.* [Recorded by] KC and The Sunshine Band. Epic.

[8] Richie, L. (1983). *Hello.* Motown.

[9] Nitzsche, J., Sainte-Marie, B., & Jennings, W. (1982). *Up Where We Belong.* [Recorded by] Cocker, J., & Warnes, J. On *An Officer and a Gentleman.* [Medium of recording]. Island.

[10] Pegler, T. (1972). *Organ Hoedown.* Jackson Music Limited.

[11] Hudson, W., Mills, I., & De Lange, E. (1933). *Moonglow* [First Recorded by] Venuti, J.

[12] Anson, J. (1977). *The Amityville Horror.* Prentice Hall.

[13] Branson, R. (2018). [*Twitter*] 24 January 2018.

Chapter 4

M301! Here We Come

'When you don't know how to get to where you want to be ... just trust you will be guided step by step. Hold your vision ... no one knew how to get to the moon ... but they made it. You'll learn how to get there one step at a time.'

~ Michelle Townsend

Now, you might think what on earth is this title for a chapter of a book! It is in fact the number of the very first mobile phone I purchased back in 1995; a Motorola which was introduced for the Mercury One2One network. Sounds like something out of space, doesn't it! Little did I realise when I purchased the phone where this journey would take me, and oh my goodness, was it going to be a journey! A journey of communication, or should I say lack of. Yes, we can communicate! No, we can't communicate! The frustration of the carrot being dangled, then taken away, was, in hindsight, a strong metaphor for the roller-coaster journey that was about to unfold.

In **May 1995**, Karl and I become aware that people were buying mobile phones. They were starting to appear more in shops with a choice of phones to choose from…interesting.

However, they were like carrying a house brick around with you! I mean how convenient (inconvenient!!) I had also heard that the signal wasn't that fantastic. You had to go to certain areas where signals were being emitted to use the phones. Was this really worth it?

We happened to walk into an electrical store, whilst shopping one weekend and spotted a lovely phone. Nowadays it would be like a brick, but at the time it wasn't; it seemed quite a nice size to what we had previously heard about! We asked some questions about how it worked and were told signals were getting much better. We discussed the matter, and decided it was possibly a good idea and worth investing in. I was driving a lot as a mobile music teacher working late nights. Winter nights were dark ... so .... with what seemed a great idea, we walked out of the shop with a Motorola M301 phone and a tariff to pay for each month. Good investment, I thought at the time... feeling quite excited and pleased with myself - being one of the limited people that now owned a 'Mobile Phone' GREAT! I felt quite techy, up to date and with it!

We got it home, set the charger up and left the mobile phone charging for a few hours. Once fully charged, we started to try it out. To my disappointment, there was no signal whatsoever ... 'ooh!!' I kept trying to dial out and nothing ... absolutely nothing!

At that time, there still wasn't full coverage over the UK. Mobile phone masts were slowly being erected with the main areas being London, Manchester and Birmingham. After ringing the mobile phone company and questioning this, we realised that it would eventually work better over time, as coverage would slowly be improved and expanded. Rather expensive to say the least when you aren't getting the full service!

In the weeks that followed, I made a visit to Manchester. I drove my sister, her friend, and Mom to see the band 'Take That' in concert. 'Great!' I thought. 'Now was my chance to try out my new mobile phone.' After parking up and sorting ourselves out, I checked to see if the phone was picking any signals up. The signal was brilliant in Manchester, I couldn't believe it! Everywhere I walked, the signal was there. The phone calls were brilliant too. It was great to be mobile and communicate without using a good ole red telephone box. I called both my husband and my dad. It was exciting - finally my mobile worked! It was good to hear their voices really clear on the other end of the line. With all the excitement, I called them several times in different areas of the city, just to prove it still worked. Signals seemed to be better along the motorways. Mobile phone masts were being installed on main routes where they were expanding the coverage from.

Slowly the signals got better and better, continually improving. I never really noticed any problems at this point; I just got on with the convenience of having the phone. I loved it!

Eventually the coverage in our area improved and you could use the phone for most calls. The younger generation just take mobiles for granted. It's become a main and normal part of our lives now; it's part of the furniture, part of us.

A Way Will Be Found

Back then, the gradual rollout of mobile phones and their masts, which would allow the communication that we now have, was taking its time, slowly taking shape. Just like we all must learn to communicate with each other with our different frequencies, perceptions and understandings. The designers who created this technology didn't know what they know now. We develop over time, technology develops over time; learning to communicate takes time and practice. If we can work and process life from a place of frequency and *'energy'*, it can be a game changer - life-changing in fact - just like a mobile phone connects via a set of numbers through frequency. **'Energy'** is everywhere; everything is **'energy!'** When you send a text message from your mobile, do you see all the letters releasing themselves out the end of the phone, flying through the air, to land in the other persons phone? No. So how does the message get sent? Frequency, wavelength, *'energy!'*

It's the same with ideas. When we take on a new project, we tend not to know how we are going to get to the final destination. We just have an idea of the outcome we want. That idea has *'energy'*. Rather than doubting, feeling that it can't be done, or not knowing how, trust you will be guided step by step. We don't need to know the whole journey - each step will guide us to the next. Ideas will flow ... you'll try this ... you'll try that ... you'll learn from your mistakes. Use them as your guidance. We are surrounded by so many things, showing us how we develop over time. Just like the technology of mobile phones has developed, we also develop, but we forget to honour this within ourselves. It's not necessarily something we consider. We don't always know how we are going to do something or approach something, but in that moment, we make the decision *'a way will be found.'* Guidance steps in, the *'energy'* around it starts to awaken, attracting other options. What's important here is to remember to enjoy the journey! What's the point of doing it otherwise? Learn to communicate with the creativity!

Most people that know me well, know I talk about thoughts. Everything is first created by a thought. 'Thoughts create things'. Thoughts have *'energy'*. Just like a designer designs the draft for a new building from his thoughts which he puts down on paper. It's important to remember that most things in life are also created this way, just like the development of mobile phones over the years. Even the seat that you are sitting on started that way. Someone had to think that thought in their mind to come up with the idea, the shape, the size, the textures and colours chosen for it. We have a habit of forgetting this for ourselves. We create ourselves. Yes, there are many things beyond our control, but we attract all of it. You are a frequency emitter just like a mobile phone mast. You set your frequency. Whatever your frequency is set too, you'll attract things on that same wavelength. The same goes with getting on with certain people or not. There lies the old saying ... *'Oh, we are on the same wavelength.'* According to Sydney J. Harris (originally misattributed to George Bernard Shaw) ... *"Life is not about finding yourself; it's about creating yourself."*[1]

When we look at life in general, we just flow through life on autopilot. Thinking that things just happen and fall into place just because they do. Ninety-five per cent of our life is subconscious/unconscious. If we take a deeper look into how life flows, we do indeed have a lot of power in each moment. Life propels us forward in remarkable ways. Driving our choices forward in the way we are focused. You get what you are focused on. Just like sending that message to a friend, we have quite a lot of control over it, more than we realise; you are sending out that frequency, that 'energy'. When we stop and think about how we are going to approach life's challenges and paths, usually we can choose what feels right to us in that moment to step forward, connecting into feeling good. So, what if we are trying to achieve a direction and we have no idea where to start? Where do we go with it? The thought of even starting new ventures totally freaks us out! What happens then?

Use the unknown. The fact that you have initially thought about a possibility creates the first step, the first thought. One thought leads to another. Acknowledge that possibility. If we can make the decision to just go for it and persist, things start to fall into place, each step leading to the next step; it propels us along the way. Even though we feel we aren't moving forward, we are. Allow the vulnerability to inspire you, create the adventure. It's just a process which we must allow; foster a feeling of trust that we will be guided along that path. No-one knew how to do anything to start with. Look at life around you in great detail - everything develops, everything creates, every person gains wisdom on their journey. Seize the unknown. Use it for personal growth, allow it to ignite your inner desires. Take some time to stop and think about how all things develop and change over time. YOU ARE NOT STATIC! You are always moving forward. This isn't something we consider daily; we all get drawn into our daily chores. When you become more aware of that development, you start to realise you are a work of art in progress too! Draw strength from your past experiences to create new ones. Remember to honour that! It's important! Learn to communicate with YOU! It's amazing what you can create! Emit the frequency of that!

References:

[1] 1969 April 18, Record-Gazette, Strictly Personal by Sydney J. Harris (Syndicated), Quote Page 1, Column 10, Banning, California. (Newspapers_com) https://quoteinvestigator.com

Chapter 5

Momma World

Stop and take a moment to appreciate what you've achieved ... how far you have come. It's not a race ... it's a journey. Remember to savour each moment along the way. You are AMAZING!!'

~ Michelle Townsend

The day you give birth to your first-born changes your life forever. I can distinctly remember thinking; gosh, I have this wonderful little human being that depends on me for everything right now. Life will never be the same again. The sheer love and protection that oozes out of you appears from the deepest part of you. It's indescribable.

February 1998, we were blessed with our first son, Aaron. It was a reasonable birth. I had, in fact, been in labour for two weeks experiencing contractions, but nothing. I had slept on the settee in our lounge for those last few weeks of my pregnancy. We laugh about it now; I broke the settee! I was admitted to hospital to be induced; I'd gone 12 days over my due date.

Whilst checking on the monitors, the nurse said ... *"Michelle you are having contractions all over the place!"*

I replied ... *"I know, I've been like it for two weeks!"*

"You've been in labour for two weeks Michelle! Let's get this kick started properly."

After checking me over and attempting to break my waters, the midwife realised I had none! It was, what they call a dry birth. The concern was had my waters broken in the weeks before - with risk of possible infection? But everything seemed fine. As soon as the relevant medications that were required to induce me were applied, the contractions kicked in big time. They obviously just needed a bit of a nudge; either that, or Aaron couldn't make his mind up when he was going to show up! Twelve hours later baby Townsend arrived! It took a couple of days for Karl and I to decide on a name.

Considering the birth was a dry birth, it had gone well, apart from me requiring a few stitches. I was stitched back up there and then, with baby in arms; no anaesthetic.

"You've just gone through all that pain of giving birth Michelle, so a few stitches won't hurt you!"

A 7lb 8oz baby can be a bit hard going! Five days later, after blood pressure issues, concerns of a baby being taken from the hospital (thankfully the baby was found) and being extra alert faffing about with alarms on babies' ankles which kept falling off, we returned home - completely mesmerised with this new bundle of joy that had entered our lives.

I loved being a mom. So many happy moments, a laugh a minute - but this fear of lifts and enclosed spaces suddenly became more obvious. When having to use lifts with Aaron's pushchair, I was refusing to enter them. It had to be addressed! Had this fear linked all the way back to being stuck in that lift with my mom when I was 2? Was my subconscious trying to protect me? By using glass lifts, I eventually reprogrammed this *'fear'*. There are certain lifts I still refuse to enter nowadays, but it has improved.

Karl and I had 4 years and 4 months with Aaron before our second child was born. We all remember September 11th, 2001 - the 9/11 devastation at the World Trade Centre in New York, also our wedding anniversary. A few days earlier I discovered I was expecting again. Karl and I were both so excited. Both our pregnancies had been planned; fortunately I got caught straight away with both; we were very blessed. Pictures of the Twin Towers in New York were beginning to fill our TV screens, bringing complete shock and disbelief. Everyone remembers what they were doing in their lives when such devastating things happen. The subconscious creates an anchor, just like when hearing a song that instantly takes you back to a distant memory. It's these high emotional links that create that strong anchor for us. It's why I remember that day so well. My immediate thoughts at the time were ... *'Why on earth would I choose to bring another child into this world with such devastation occurring?'* I know we shouldn't think like that but sometimes it just can't be helped. My instinct was to protect that wonderful little new being inside of me. It was bizarre really, but those thoughts were in fact happening in my head, my inner voice.

June 2002, we were blessed with another healthy boy. Here we were again - my due date passed, going over exactly 12 days, just like Aaron. I was booked in to be induced, but thankfully on the morning I was due to be admitted into hospital, my contractions became regular, so off we trundled to the hospital. Around 7 hours later and in the midst of a World Cup match, Ethan was born - an 8lb 7oz baby. Not that I can remember much about the match whilst pushing through the contractions (probably why Ethan loves football so much!). The birth flowed, my body taking over; it still amazes me to this day. This time my waters broke; gosh they did come like a tidal wave! Unlike Aaron's birth. Just as the last big push was about to happen, everything seemed to stop! Ethan's head had crowned. I could feel his head. We could see he had dark hair.

It was literally one last push; we were waiting for the next contraction.

"Next one and you'll have your baby Michelle!" ... were the midwife's words, but we seemed to be waiting forever.

Baby was in the birth canal, so really needed to come out. Then suddenly, the final contraction, and after one final superwoman push, Ethan was born. It was a concerning few minutes and once again I had to be stitched back together. I'd been ripped to smithereens. Giving birth to an 8lb 7oz baby when you're quite small can be a bit hard on your bits down there! It took at least half an hour to sort me out, but all was good again. Both Karl and I felt extremely blessed.

The boys enjoyed many happy moments. We did lots of things as a family, especially our holidays in our touring caravan, venturing off to Wales, Euro Disney - France, Holland and Belgium to name but a few. As parents, we gave our boys the best we could, trying out different hobbies and interests along the way. Encouraging them to experience those different choices and options. They were both amazing swimmers. Aaron especially took to competitive swimming with a swimming club in our local area. He was known for his butterfly stroke. The club always put him in for this heat in the competitions. Training was most evenings and sometimes even early mornings. Competitions took up most weekends, travelling here and there. It took up so much time. Both boys loved fishing with their dad, enjoying many fishing trips, including sea fishing. There were many happy times spent at the fisheries by our caravan in Wales. Along with all this Aaron, Ethan and I took up karate, successfully gaining our blue belts before deciding to stop lessons because of my health - we just had too much going on. But it was music that was going to be their mainstay. Music seemed to be their first love too - Aaron a percussionist and Ethan a saxophonist. Both started piano lessons with me at an early age and continued music lessons through school.

Aaron chose drum kit and percussion - Ethan chose saxophone. It was me that really wanted to learn drums in the beginning. Karl bought a kit to get me started, but it was all three of us that ended up having lessons from an amazing drummer called Daniel Hayward. I even got a distinction in my 'Grade 3' drums! Piano had triggered and fired up both boys' interests and I went on to teach them both theory of music. Eventually, Aaron continued his drumming and swimming and Ethan his piano and saxophone. Their private teachers worked wonders with them! Along with Daniel for drum kit, Julian Powell helped Aaron tremendously with tuned percussion. A wonderful lady called Madge helped Ethan with piano. We needed that outside ritual as sometimes it's not easy teaching your own children. It can turn into ... *'Oh, we will do your lesson tomorrow scenario.'* We needed the outside stability. We just had so much fun!

The natural protective instinct that comes from becoming a parent is so strong, it just exudes from you. Like all toddlers, both Aaron and Ethan had their tumbles. We've all had them. Some stay imprinted in your mind. Aaron was around two when he lost his footing and tripped and fell in our hallway towards the stairs. He hit his cheekbone, just by his eye, on the corner of the wooden banister. The dent that appeared in his cheek will stay in my mind forever. Thankfully, he was ok and never damaged his eye.

Ethan always had a habit of falling over. Both Karl and I were always on tender hooks because we knew what he was like. He would fall over his own shadow if we let him! Ethan also had an eye injury whilst we were away on holiday in Holland in our touring caravan. He scraped his eye on a bush, scratching right across his pupil. We managed to stay calm. Our family must have had an eye thing going on! There was Wi-Fi on the site - albeit the dinosaur version - which I seemed reasonably ok with at the time. Karl managed to find information on what to do and Ethan's injury healed the next day. I had put mom's special healing hands over his eye to take it away. It reassured the 4-year-old Ethan that it was going to get better; there lies a subconscious belief! The worst fall Ethan experienced was coming off his skateboard and hitting his pelvis on the curb outside our house.

Because he had so many silly falls, we just said ... *"You'll be fine, rub it better."*

Half an hour later, whilst we were preparing dinner, Ethan fainted and collapsed on our kitchen floor, hitting his head. You can imagine the response and panic! After coming round, Ethan started hyperventilating and panicking and an emergency trip to the hospital followed. For several years after, Ethan responded differently to any pain related injury. As a child he was fearless; it never bothered him to fall or overcome an injury. But this experience changed his perspective subconsciously - not liking hospitals or being treated for injuries, it really left a mark on the deeper part of his mind. Fainting spells occurred in those situations because his mind now thought it had to protect him by taking his focus away from pain. It's amazing how the subconscious creates this protection for us through our life experiences.

Becoming a mom has been my proudest achievement in my life so far. My boys are the best things I've ever created in my whole life! Life completely changes in a split second, the blessings, happy times, responsibilities, new communications and friends, but also the trials and tribulations of being a parent. We all worry, don't we? We want to protect our children completely. I've achieved many things in life, things I never thought would have been possible for me - including writing the book you now hold in your hand. How the bloody hell did I do that? But I did!! Out of everything, nothing tops or even comes near to becoming a mom; that is by far my proudest most amazing achievement ever!

I built up a powerful protection for my boys, hiding away what was really happening deep inside me. I didn't want the boys knowing or even understanding what EHS was. I didn't want them to create it for themselves. I knew how programming worked. I was starting to understand how the mind worked. I wanted to protect them. That became my fear for them. Symptoms started developing further. A phone call one night was about to create a turning point in my life that I would never have dreamed I would experience! I don't know where I found the strength that was hiding the weakness within. Looking back, it was the start of cancer within my body, but it was being masked by my focus and thoughts on Electromagnetic Hypersensitivity.

A Way Will Be Found

Where does this strength come from? This strength to keep everything alright. Is it that place of unconditional love? We all put protection barriers up throughout our life, but who in the end are we protecting? Are we protecting our loved ones or ourselves? We must ask ourselves those questions. Even though we may be a parent, have family members and amazing friends, it is so important to be there for ourselves, to honour what's right and not right within us. If we are not there for ourselves, how on earth can we be there for the most important people around us? It all starts with YOU! It's not selfish to be there for YOU!

Becoming a mom made me realise many things, changes in perspective especially. We all care about our loved ones and closest friends, but being a parent is different. The love for our parents is different to the love we share with our partners. It's a different kind of love for our friends. But the love that oozes from you when you become a parent is the love of sheer protection, unconditional love. You just want to wrap your children up in cotton wool, not wanting them to get hurt. Protecting them in every way possible. It never changes as they get older. Situations change and there's something new or different to worry about. You must learn to let them go, allowing them to become the best person they can be, hoping that you've instilled enough understanding, respect and kind-heartedness in them to help support them through life. Afterall, we never own our children. They are their own unique person. We are just the vehicles that brought them forward into physical form. If you think you own your children, it's wise to change that perspective as soon as you can, for it can only hinder relationships. No-one owns anyone! We just share our lives together on this journey of life.

Being a teacher and working with children over many years, I learnt how to deal with different situations, different personalities. That part of my life helped when becoming a parent. But there's so much more you learn as a parent. Obviously, there's no manual on parenting; it comes from what's been instilled in you from beliefs, experiences, perceptions and our programming.

Reverse psychology is especially interesting; if done correctly, it can create empowerment. I often chuckle to myself when becoming aware of using it subtlety. When we mollycoddle our children, we are in fact disempowering them; not allowing them to become the true person that they are. Remember the 'inner child?' Mollycoddling and doing everything for our children takes away their strength to become the best they can be. Yes, we need to support and guide young children, but also need to allow them to make their own choices and decisions; let them get stuck into life and show them how to do that, creating independence. That's true parenting! Ask your children what they want, what they like, and you'll bring out their true personality, their true 'inner child.'

Aaron's drum lessons were going well, but there came a time when the practice started waning off. Karl and I mentioned to him that it was important to maintain practice to get better, but to no avail. Aaron would do a little bit of practice here and there. It was decided that if things didn't improve, lessons would have to stop. It was a waste of money if Aaron wasn't going to use his drum lessons to gain full potential from them. Of course, Aaron didn't want this to happen, but his competitive swimming took up so much time. So, like my parents had done with me back when I was 17, we suggested he made a choice. Swimming or music! We threatened to stop music lessons so many times. Thankfully, practice picked up. In hindsight, that would have been terribly criminal after what he has now achieved with his music.

After transferring from school to private tuition, Ethan had a fantastic saxophone teacher called Joanne Naylor who did him extremely proud. Joanne was, in fact, one of my original pupils whom I had taught electronic organ and theory to back when she was 5. She later studied saxophone. Ethan wasn't putting the time in either drums or saxophone. It was decided to stop the drum lessons and threaten the same with the saxophone. Ethan didn't like it, thinking we wouldn't go through with it. He loved his saxophone. Karl took over Ethan's saxophone lessons for a month. Every time the lesson was due, Ethan would get upset that his dad was now having his lesson. He hated it! Amazingly, Ethan started practising his saxophone. This decision could have backfired completely, but we had to do something. From that point on, you couldn't get Ethan off his saxophone, promising he would practise from there on in. Reverse psychology fully places the decision with the other person. It wasn't for us as parents to decide: we just put things in place for Ethan to make that choice, that decision. We never wanted him to stop, my heart was breaking inside, it was so hard, hoping that it would trigger a response within him to continue. Thankfully it did!

We all want help, support and guidance from people close to us, but they can only give advice from their perspective and experiences. They are not living our life - we are. They can't make our choices and decisions; they can only give a perspective on it. Usually, we find the most important aspect that holds us back in making decisions is 'fear'. We use excuses for not doing something because we don't feel good enough or believe we can't achieve it. It's our personal protection barrier, coming from our past experiences, running at a subconscious level. If someone really wants to do something but is making excuses through fear or just can't be bothered, they won't like it if you agree with them; they want you to guide them, they want advice to reassure them. There can come a certain amount of wanting attention here, we are all only human - it's a human trait - just like it's easier to do negative thinking. People want you to feel sorry for them, and it's no good disagreeing with that because it's true. Just admit it! You'll soon shift away from it!

So, what do we mean by reverse psychology? Agree with what a person says, turn it on its head. 'If that's what you want to do, then leave it, don't go for it.' Or ... 'Yes, I agree with you, carry on,' even if you don't. It's not lying to them; it's placing the decision completely into their hands. Sometimes it's the best guidance you can give. Everyone must find their own truth, communicate with themselves, find what feels good. By being aware of not being true to ourselves, stopping ourselves from doing something and not stepping forward, completely changes the decision and the choices; making that move to create deep down what you really want. You give people that awareness by highlighting it with your response. Empower them! It's interesting to watch. You can see instantly that it kills the attention they are seeking. It really does kick them into deciding for themselves. It also makes people realise that they are in control of their own life - no one else can make the decision - no one else can live their life. Yes, ask and get advice but it's what you do with the advice afterwards that makes the difference.

I have especially experienced this with my writing over the last few years. I was fearful of not being good enough, not using 'BIG' impressive words - as I call them - when I write, going round in circles. Making excuses not to write to get out of the embarrassment. It's took me a long time to put that aside, a very long time. I now practise the approach that if I can help just one person to look at life differently, I've done my job.

As I write this chapter, it's July 2023. I'm sitting in the sunshine at the back of P&O Iona, enjoying the sounds of the swell created from the ship's propellers. It's our last sea day before returning to Southampton after cruising to Norway. This whole chapter has been written on my phone in notes on Iona, just like many chapters or parts of my book. 'A way will be found'... moving from 'fear' to 'freedom' if you look and search for it within.

Michelle Townsend

Chapter 6

Starting to Notice the Effects

'Think of yourself as a big energy bubble floating about.
Whatever energy you are emitting ...
you will attract the same frequency back.'

~ Michelle Townsend

In the years that followed, this powerful statement from Darryl Anka (originally misattributed to Einstein), was one that I became to understand as extremely true ...

'Everything is energy and that's all there is to it.
Match the frequency of the reality you want, and you cannot help but get that reality.
It can be no other way.
This is not philosophy. This is physics.'[1]

~ Darryl Anka

Life carried on pretty much as normal for a while. I enjoyed being a mom. I continued enjoying my work as a private music teacher, working from home. On becoming a mom,

I cut my hours of work down by half to get a balance and allow me to enjoy the boys growing up.

In October 1998, after giving birth to Aaron in February, I became surrounded by a new set of friends, all of us new moms. One evening, I made a phone call from my mobile phone to a friend for a chat. I had a certain number of free minutes at the time, so thought it was a good idea to use them. I remember being on the phone quite a while with the conversation going on over half an hour. Suddenly, I noticed my battery was going flat. Not knowing what I know now, (NOTE: never use your phone while it's plugged in and charging), I plugged my phone into the power supply and carried on chatting. I noticed the phone getting a little warm but carried on regardless. By the time I had finished the phone call, I felt a little bit of discomfort at the side of my head where I had held the phone. It felt a bit numb, but I thought nothing of it. Maybe the heat from the charging was to blame.

Over the next few months, I started to notice a sensation by my ear and side of my head when I used the phone. I started to question and link the sensations with the phone. Initially, I dismissed it, but when it continued to happen, I became more and more aware that it wasn't just a coincidence.

May 1999. Having booked a caravan holiday to Croyde Bay, Devon, I distinctly remember sitting in the car travelling to our destination feeling preoccupied … I was concerned and thinking about this mobile phone. *'Mmm … I wonder … is this phone really doing this to me? Is it really causing sensations in my head?'* I was paying over £48 a month for the tariff at the time. It was a lot to be spending, especially if I couldn't use the phone in the way I wanted to. By now I was on my second phone, plus Karl now had one.

I kept asking him … *"Does the phone make your head this …"* and *"Does the phone make your head that …?"*

One day, whilst sitting in the caravan, I took it upon myself to ring my phone suppliers, explaining to them that the phone was making my head hurt.

I asked them … *"Does anyone else have this problem?"*

But of course, they weren't going to admit that were they? To be honest they must have thought I had lost the plot and was a weird freak asking questions like that. Most people reacted that way when I mentioned it. I tried so hard, persisting with the phone. Of course, I loved the convenience of it. What a fantastic gadget. On the other hand, I was getting so frustrated and became frightened of it. I couldn't bear the phone by my head. I was experiencing numbness, tingling and sharp pains in my head, which eventually started to work their way down into my arms. I found myself not using the phone or avoiding it.

Finally, one day my father-in-law said, *"Are you using your phone now?"*

"I haven't tried it for a while." I replied.

He tried to ring me on my mobile. I answered. Then, within a split second of putting it by my head to answer, I had such a surge of pain in my head and arm, I literally threw the phone out of my hand in shock!

With great disappointment and frustration, I eventually changed to a 'Pay as You Go' tariff as I wasn't using enough data to justify the rather large amount I was paying per month. I eventually switched to just texting people. This was around the time when texting wasn't that popular. I felt safer just texting. I hadn't got to put the phone by my head. It just goes to show how much I used it, only costing me around £20/30 a year! I carried on like this for a couple of years and things didn't seem too bad. I lost interest in my phone, just accepting that I couldn't use a mobile phone by my head.

As our youngest son began to grow up, we started noticing things changing with my health. I had breast fed both my babies, my youngest one being more successful than the first.

It was time to stop when he reached 11 months old, as I had the wonderful pleasure of him biting me, so it was getting rather painful... ouch! Reluctantly, I decided to stop, as he was going to do me an injury if I wasn't careful! But as soon as I stopped breast feeding, my health seemed to suffer a little. Silly little things like when I put my contact lenses in, my eyes would start to react. The whites of my eyes would swell, so I had to stop wearing the contact lenses. I also noticed that I became very tired easily. I suffered from low emotions, feeling low and tearful. I was losing weight very quickly and went extremely thin.

One afternoon we were sitting talking to Karl's mom and dad. They were telling us about the wonderful time they had just had on their cruise and showing us photos. As I was listening, I started to feel overwhelmingly upset, thinking ... *'I'm never going to be able to go on a cruise ship because of all the radar and frequencies on them.'* I started to think all sorts of things around these frequencies. Stopping me doing so much. One thought led to another. I ended up taking myself off to the toilet so I could hide my feelings and try to sort myself out. This was becoming my life. And yet now, after all that worry of going on a cruise ship because of the radar, I'm writing parts of my book on one!

Around 2007, planning had been put forward to our local council for a mobile phone mast to be erected in a field near our street. I went into major melt down! Sitting in our caravan on our drive, I was discussing it with my father-in-law and Karl.

"We must petition against it! I can't have a mobile phone mast by our house. It's going to make me ill!"

I probably drove them mad with it, but thankfully the mobile phone mast didn't come to fruition.

Electrical sensitivity can create a lot of negative emotions and frustration in the person who is experiencing it. You feel like you are a weird being and people look at you as such and laugh when you tell them what you feel. They can't comprehend it.

"Don't be so silly - mobile phones and Wi-Fi won't do that to you, I don't have any symptoms!"

I knew people didn't necessarily mean it; I just think they didn't know how to respond, to be honest. People can be very inconsiderate and do not understand the situation from your perspective, so they do and say things that can be very hurtful without realising. I had many instances of this. People really didn't know how to react to the situation, because there's no physical symptoms to see. I had to release these conversations from my head and forgive people. Hanging onto any negativity was not going to do me any good and was sure to dig me deeper. I was feeling **really** angry and frustrated about it.

I started to put up resistance to fight my corner ... *"Yes, it does exist! Why don't you believe me?"*

I realise now that I was just convincing myself even further, thus creating more noticeable symptoms. I had to do the decent thing for myself and just agree with people! Again, not speaking up, or voicing my opinion, not being true to myself. Surprise, surprise! I experienced loneliness on a grand scale. I felt like I couldn't join in with what everyone else was doing because of being bombarded by the EMFs wherever I went. Although we always had to consider where we were going to protect me, my family never ever judged me through all of this. They really didn't know how to deal with it, but they were very thoughtful and tried not to talk about it too much. They supported me as best they could, which I will always be truly grateful for.

It's interesting that in all the years of experiencing the effects of EHS, I never read a single book about it - there aren't, in fact, many of them. Although, I do now find that awareness of EHS is being highlighted more. All along I kept backing away from that. I felt I didn't need to know too much detail about possible chemical and physical changes. With hindsight, I now know that this was the correct route for me. 'We get what we focus on'. There were no influences from anywhere other than what I had read briefly on the world wide web. The most research I had done and read about was from the 'Powerwatch. org'[2] website - which has been continually updated over the years. There isn't a lot out there. I can only speak from my own experience here, from me as an individual. If you are reading this book and thinking 'yes' that sounds just like me, then read on. When we change our perspective, our approach and thought processes towards illness, it can change our experience.

EHS, for me, I believe was a problem with communication. On an energetic level, my body was responding to my deep-seated emotions, beliefs and perceptions of life. It seemed to create a barrier, preventing me from living life normally, keeping me away from life. I truly believe that it is our bodies' way of protecting us. Not having to face situations or communicate. This truly begins in the mind from our beliefs and perceptions. The question is ... 'Why was I experiencing these responses? What was creating the pain and the feelings?' These feelings were stopping me from communicating with people. But why? Had all of this appeared because I was shy, finding it hard to communicate, not allowing myself to speak up? Was it my body's way of trying to protect me from being in those situations? Keeping me away. It was all very bizarre.

For many years before my experience with EHS and Hodgkin's Lymphoma, I always had to be very careful of bath products. I still do to this day. I have to psych myself up to try certain soaps, shower gels and make-up products, in case of the hassle of dealing with a reaction. Hypoallergenic doesn't mean anything, not a single bit! Products can be as hypoallergenic and as expensive as you wish, it doesn't stop reactions; they can even be worse. I knew what suited me and kept with that knowledge, yet I've always been perfectly fine with scented perfumes and eau de toilette. I especially love my 'Jo Malone'[3] ones now.

So, when I realised I was experiencing EHS, I did just a little bit of research on Powerwatch. I found that other people who were experiencing EHS also had chemical sensitivity. Maybe that was why I had problems with certain bath products? I accepted this and never thought any more about it until the diagnosis of Hodgkin's Lymphoma. If I tended to be chemically reactive to certain products and was to receive chemotherapy treatment lasting 6 Months, how was my body going to react? I had this thought, that I could be chemically sensitive, at the back of my mind - was I chemically sensitive? It really makes you question the possibilities here. In time, I came to realise that I did not believe I was chemically sensitive. If I was, I would have found myself in a right state from receiving the chemotherapy drugs. My beliefs about chemical sensitivity being linked to Electromagnetic Hypersensitivity don't exist. My experience suggests otherwise.

The symptoms of EHS can vary from person to person. Symptoms can be subtle, harsh, or gradually appear slowly. I noticed my first symptoms 24 years ago. Looking back, mine was a very gradual build up, while others just become very sensitive straight away. It's very different for everyone.

Listed below are the symptoms in the order I experienced them. Others' experiences may be slightly different ...

- Warmth on the side of my head when using a mobile phone developing into tingling and pain the side of my head.
- Loss of concentration.
- Tiredness and dizziness.

I then noticed the same symptoms when using digital house phones. These symptoms then developed into ...

- Tingling and pain in my arms and body when in contact with Wi-Fi.
- Shaking all over the body and nearly collapsing on the floor. The only way I can describe it, is it was like I was resonating with the frequencies.
- Feeling sick, loss of co-ordination.
- Tinnitus in ears, very high pitch ringing all the time.

After removing myself from the items, the symptoms eventually lapsed and then I felt as fit as a fiddle again. Other symptoms included ...

- Sore eyes after using the computer.
- Feeling drained and tired after using the computer.
- Dry eyes, pain all round eye area, eyes feeling swollen.
- Pain in the back.

Again, after an interval of rest from the above equipment, I'd feel fine!

Until **October 2007,** I was managing the sensitivity extremely well. I had it under control, adapting my life around it. Adjusting things such as only using my mobile phone for texting, going back to corded house phones, avoiding Wi-Fi (which was controllable back then whereas it isn't now). We even had to consider choosing caravan sites that were free from Wi-Fi connections. EHS affected every part of our lives. The more Wi-Fi appeared, the more I started to notice symptoms on a regular basis. The physical symptoms seemed to take over and I experienced things such as ...

- Breathing problems and pains in chest.
- Heart palpitations.

- High D-dimers in my blood (mine reached 5000! Apparently, the normal level is around 220 - 500ng/mL, around 600, it's possible you have a blood clot or a major infection somewhere). Anything above 1000 could be a possible pulmonary embolism. We are not sure whether this was to do with my later cancer diagnosis in January 2010. Nothing was done with the results of the D-dimers, as nothing could be found at the time, so we will never really know. I had scans to try and find blood clots, but nothing proved to show in the results.

I became aware of articles about EMFs causing blood cancer and of newspaper articles regarding issues with cars. My symptoms got incredibly worse when we changed our car in October 2007. Within a day of driving our new car, my symptoms seemed to just tip me right over the edge; the electrics in the car were now affecting me. Luckily our older 4 x 4 (11 years old at the time) was fine so I could still go out, but in the new car I experienced ...

- Near Fainting while driving.
- Sever pain in my head, arms, chest and body.
- Stiffness and limited movement in my body; muscles feeling knotted and tense.
- Incredible tiredness and lack of energy.
- Different organs in my body would start to resonate with the frequencies at different times causing pain.

Then all other electrical items started to become a real problem. It seemed like everything electrical was affecting me. I started struggling teaching. I would dread starting work because I knew I was going to be in agony for hours. I would sit at the side of my pupil at the keyboard, concentrating on teaching and keep telling myself to 'relax and breathe'. *You've taught for many years without this response so you can do it again,'* I'd say to myself. It became an affirmation that just rolled around in my head without me even thinking about it. This just shows that if you repeat something enough, it runs automatically, just like learning a piece of music. I used to calm myself down if I felt myself getting frustrated; *'relax and breathe', 'relax and breathe'* over and over.

I was trying so hard to create a change from this experience, but only created more stress. *'How can I live in a world where I can't get on with electricity? How am I going to function? What's my life going to be like in the future?'* I had all sorts of thoughts running through my head, day after day, week after week, month after month, it was hard going and used up a lot of my energy. EHS is very draining, not only from the reactions, but from trying to deal with the emotions that come with it. I even worried if there was going to come a time where I would no longer be able to work.

I distinctly remember sitting teaching on my electronic instruments, and even though I had the communication of the pupil and interaction, I felt like I was in a bubble of loneliness, dealing with pain, emotion, frustration, upset, that went on and on. That's what it felt like.

I dread to think how many lessons I taught in agony! It was certainly a great deal. Pupils were understanding though. I didn't admit it to everyone, for the fear of being looked at like this mad woman who is allergic to electricity! I'd seen people's responses before. *'How can you be allergic to electricity?'* I only told people who I knew wouldn't judge me. It was at this point in my life that I was so limited as to what I could do. I was so frustrated and was losing the will to live. This was the turning point for me. A dear friend of mine, who was also a healer, had been helping me keep my symptoms under control over the last 6 or 7 years using natural remedies; she was now suggesting try hypnotherapy.

So, what can affect you? For people who are not electrically sensitive, the list below will seem hilarious. However, people who are electrically sensitive, you will associate with this list straight away.

Look really closely at the list, from a non-sufferer's point of view, thinking about the life you lead and especially about which of these items you use and how much in a day. This will make you realise how an electrically sensitive person's life can be affected so dramatically. Put yourself in a position of what you do and then run your day with this in mind.

Items or equipment, which may affect you include ...

- Mobile phones.
- Mobile phone masts.
- Wi-Fi.
- Digital house phones.
- Computers.
- Televisions - old and the new LCDs, LEDs etc.
- Modern cars - even without Bluetooth and Sat-Navs.
- Anything Bluetooth.
- Satellite Navigation systems.
- Iron.
- Hair dryer.
- Household electrical items (lamps, lights, etc.).
- From my own experience, my electronic organ, keyboard and electronic piano.

Basically, think of anything electrical. It varies with each sufferer and this list is far from exhaustive.

***

It's a Wednesday morning 31st of March 2021 and I've just finished teaching an online lesson. I'm sitting at my electric piano, my computer in front of me, my mobile phone next to me and I'm completely comfortable. Back in the day, that would not have been possible at all! I also have a Wi-Fi router in my music room that my computer connects to. I also have wired internet - which I only use because it's more stable. I certainly don't use it to sway away from Wi-Fi! In fact, the Wi-Fi is still switched on. It's there for when I move around the house and move my computer to another room.

During my period of sensitivity, I couldn't even think about or connect to this type of situation as being an option in the future. When I think about it all now, I feel very proud of myself and what I've achieved and changed within me. Who would have thought it could have been possible? How has it been possible? Power lies within us, and we have access to it 100% of the time. It's just how we choose to use that power. I am so grateful for this understanding that I now have, which I use in all areas of my life.

***

A Way Will Be Found

We are all electromagnetic beings, whether we believe it or not. We give off a frequency from our thoughts and what we are feeling. We emit that specific frequency. Any frequencies which match those thoughts and feelings tend to show up in our experience, in the reality around us. This is known as the 'Law of Attraction', a law of the universe. If you have ever studied physics, you'll be aware of frequency and resonance. Everything in the universe resonates at its own frequency.

If we can have a deeper understanding of this scientific knowledge, we can start to create a different response and change our frequency. In turn, we can create change in our lives and the reality around us, even powerful healing - as I found out. I was about to change the effects of EHS by using my mind, my thoughts and my feelings. I was about to change the frequency and responses I was experiencing.

Physics proves that frequencies match, vibrate and resonate together or with each other.

Thoughts have frequency. One thought leads to another thought of the same frequency. We attract more of the same. It's hard not to talk about something when it is affecting you at a deeper level; you need to prove it's true. We think that by talking about something more helps us to deal with it. However, when we are thinking about a specific subject, or have a specific focus, we are much more likely to bring that into our experience, because we are giving off the frequency of that thought. I use the example of 'don't think of a *pink pig*, do think of a *pink pig*' during my hypnotherapy sessions to help people understand that it is the object of attention that creates the focus - not the 'do' or 'don't' part. Whether you 'do' or you 'don't', you are still thinking about a *'pink pig'* either way! The subconscious does not understand the difference between 'do' or 'don't' - it's the subject matter. We must start to learn that words and thoughts have power!! **'Energy!!'** By talking about the subject at hand, we are communicating with it more and bringing it closer to us. The more you talk about it, keeping a connection with it through your thoughts, the more you will find it resonating in your experience. 'Thoughts create things.' You keep it in your *'energy'* bubble. The direction of where that subject goes can be completely changed at any point in time, because the subconscious does not distinguish between past, present, or future; it just works with NOW! Time does not exist in the subconscious. This can then allow us to move forward and help heal our body from adverse responses. This includes emotions, feelings, pain and even illness.

If the subject you are talking about feels great, feels good and makes you happy, then continue; keep feeding it! Keep it resonating!! Keep talking about it! You'll find things matching the frequency you are emitting; your experience will bring forward more of what you are talking about. If the subject no longer resonates with you, feels uncomfortable, makes you unhappy, sad, ill, make a decision to let it go. Accepting what's happening or has happened can then change your thoughts around it and allow a refocus. Focus on what you want, not what you don't want! Change the way you talk about it. Some people will say ... 'Well, you are not dealing with the issue by not talking about it, it's good to talk'. Choose to say it once, get it off your chest, then refocus. Focus on the resolution, rather than the issue.

Sadly, human beings are negatively biased and find it easier to talk about negative stuff!! They love it!! They love the drama, even if they don't admit it! That's why I found it hard. I'm only human after all, but in the end I did it!! Use the adversity to create the change. If you persist, you CAN redirect your thoughts around anything! Stop the 'woe is me', stop feeling sorry for yourself, it doesn't get you anywhere. Choose to step forward in your empowerment! It's all about perspective.

My intention is, if it is possible for me to create change, then it is possible for others to also create change. After all ...

'What's possible for one, is possible for all!'[4]

~ Kelly Noonan-Gores

References:

[1]Anka, D (n.d.). Misattributed to Einstein, A. [Online] Available at:
https://www.goodreads.com/quotes/571191-everything-is-energy-and-that-s-all-there-is-to-it

[2]Powerwatch.org. Available at:
https://www.powerwatch.org.uk/ health/ sensitivity.asp

[3]Malone, J. (Est, 1990) Estée Lauder (1999)
https://www.jomalone.co.uk

[4]Gores, K.N. (2017). *Heal* [Documentary]. Available at: https://www.healdocumentary.com

Michelle Townsend

Chapter 7

Breaking Point! Journey to Hypnosis

'Your fears hold hidden gifts ... if you dare to look. Accept them, honour them, utilise them; they are a gift from the universe to strengthen your soul.'

~ Michelle Townsend

During **September 2007**, after owning my lovely white Mini Cooper for just two years, the decision was made to change it for a black Ford Focus ST. My husband had been looking for one of these makes of car for quite a while; he loved them! Karl and I happened to be looking around a Ford garage and we got talking to one of the salesmen. Changing my Mini hadn't really crossed my mind as I really did enjoy the car. Then, before we even realised it, we had ordered this new car! The car was in another part of the country, down south, so we had to wait for it to be delivered to the garage.

The decision to buy this car was mainly because it hadn't got the 'Bluetooth' connections. We couldn't add any features to the car as it had already been produced. Back in 2007, most new cars were working with Bluetooth. I didn't want those connections in my car because of the EHS I was experiencing. I wanted to be able to drive the car free from worrying about any adverse responses. I had previously ordered my Mini without Bluetooth connection for the same reasons - limiting EMF exposure.

Roughly a week later, Karl and I had the call to say that the car had arrived. We were so excited about it. We couldn't wait! But, needless to say, we had quite a disappointment. When we turned up, the car was nowhere to be seen. We were kept waiting for a considerable period of time. The salesman looked rather concerned but kept reassuring us everything was ok. When we finally got to see the car, it did look amazing. However, on closer inspection, there appeared to be a problem with the paintwork. I spotted it straight away. I'm a hawk eye for things like that - there's not much I miss! There seemed to be lots of white marks on the car, which apparently, the garage had been trying to remove - hence the long wait. The white coverings, which are put on new cars to protect them whilst in the storage yards, had damaged the paintwork in some way - almost like it had glued itself to the paintwork. The garage had done their best to remove this, but there was damage, including quite a few scratch marks, especially on the back bumper. Karl and I were so disappointed - absolutely gutted. We had to make the decision there and then to accept the car or not. As you can imagine, we didn't rush the decision.

"What are you going to do regarding the paintwork?" ... we asked.

"The paintwork will be done for you. We will even add a special coating to protect it from oxidising as it ages, free of charge."

Eventually an agreement was reached that the paintwork would be sorted professionally by the paint shop. We really wanted this car - it was at the right price and no Bluetooth! The decision was made to go ahead with the sale; we then drove it off the forecourt. Was this an omen?

In the following days, I seemed to be getting on fine with the car. I know, that's a ridiculous statement to make! But this is how it was for me. This is how I lived. However, as I was driving the car around, I started to notice a few sensations in my arms - highlighting my thoughts regarding EHS. *'Were the sensations really there? Was I thinking they were there?'* In hindsight I was. We get what we think about! By the third day, I decided to drive to Mom and Dad's and take them out for a ride to show them the new car. We ventured off to Bridgnorth, a beautiful place by the river; a good 45 minutes' drive away. As I was driving, I really started to notice these feelings in my arms. It felt like my muscles were weakening.

I mentioned this to my parents and Dad said ... *"Don't worry about it; you will be ok, try not to think about it."*

Which I did. By the time I got back home later that afternoon, I felt totally exhausted. I started to get really concerned. *'Am I going to be able to drive this new car?'* After the upset at the garage and with thoughts in my head regarding ... *'Was the paintwork a message to me not to have the car? ... Should we have refused it?'* I really was starting to get very despondent and upset. I started to feel a sense of panic. I carried on for a few more days, trying to shake it off, saying to myself ... *'Oh, it will go away, I'll be fine.'* I continued taking my youngest son to school, but each day sadly things seemed to get worse. Had the newspaper article my friend highlighted to me triggered a belief in me back then? Had the thought started subconsciously within me regarding responding to newer cars because of the new electrics in them? It was great that my friend had highlighted this and I thanked her for it at the time because it made me realise I wasn't alone with this. I found it reassuring that I wasn't the only one experiencing these symptoms. I felt that I wasn't going crazy after all! However, with the understanding I now have of the subconscious mind, it could well have been this article that created a belief within me without realising.

My husband at this point said ... *"We will just have to sell the car; we don't need to keep it."*

But that wasn't the point! I wanted this car. I loved it as a car. It was the car we had wanted for a while. My Michelle 'taurus determined head' appeared! Why should we sell a car because of the issues I was facing and ruin it for my husband? It was his absolute pride and joy!

The responses that had been building up in the few years before, I felt I had under control. Teaching on my electronic keyboard had never been an issue, nor watching TV or ironing. There were just subtle responses, until now. It's almost like I had never linked these things together, I had suddenly realised they were ALL ELECTRIC! This new car seemed to have tipped me right over the 'Electrical Sensitivity edge!' Why? What on earth was going on? It was at this point that I experienced severe pain in my arms whilst teaching on any of my electrical musical instruments. I became aware of my body responding to our TV, even sitting right back from it. Ironing would send tingling feelings running right up my arm. To sit in front of the computer was completely an absolute NO now! I really was starting to feel detached from living life, from the world. The low feelings of depression were now creeping in; they were creeping in very quickly. Much more quickly than I could ever realise.

During the time when I had my white Mini Cooper, I dealt with the initial response with the car, and it was never again a problem. The initial days of driving that car gave me slight sensations, but I addressed them and they passed within days. I never really thought about it much after that. I just enjoyed the car, but there was obviously a belief there, which I didn't realise was running deep within me. The issues with Wi-Fi, computers, mobile phone masts and mobile phones were the only things I seemed to associate and experience sensations within my body. But now it had changed to another level!

Roughly five days after collecting our new car, I had reached as far as I could go, I had a total breakdown, and I mean a total breakdown! I'd had enough! I couldn't do this anymore. I couldn't see how I could live in this world anymore. I was unable to live a normal life, meaning I couldn't use things or be by things that everyone else just took for granted. Driving my car, watching TV, using a computer, using a mobile phone, using cordless house phones - the list goes on. I was losing my communication with the world, my friends and family, in every way possible.

I had taken my youngest son to school in the Ford ST that morning. The responses whilst driving were so strong and painful, it was unbelievable. I could feel pains in my back, by my kidneys, tingling sensations running up my arms. I felt like I couldn't focus properly. My muscles felt weak, and my stomach was hurting - it was a tremendous feeling of exhaustion. I felt like I was fighting against something, and my body had gone into 'fight - flight - freeze' mode, like a rabbit in the headlights. It was this particular morning, whilst sitting in traffic on the way to school, that I had the weirdest experience, to the point I felt I was going to faint at the wheel. It was like the electrical circuits in my body went into complete turmoil. Thankfully this didn't happen, but it scared me to the point where I worried about the safety of my children. *'What if I had fainted? What if I had lost control of the car? What could have happened in a split second?'* The thoughts just kept coming. *'What if this? ... What if that?'* Believe it or not, I was managing to keep all these responses from my children, and I was doing a very good job of it! I didn't want them growing up believing electricity would hurt them. Thankfully, I got Ethan to school safely that morning, then made the return journey home. I was in agony. I cried all the way home; I couldn't wait to get back.

Once back, I went straight into the lounge where I fell to my knees, screaming and crying, rocking backwards and forwards, not knowing what to do with myself. Then, just in that moment, more powerfully than I had ever experienced them before, I had thoughts flowing through me that I really didn't want to live anymore. I wanted to end the pain I was in. I didn't want to live my life feeling trapped, not being able to go out or do things with my children, just the simple things in life. Most of all, I felt like I was causing hinderance to my family because decisions had to made around me, about what we did. The children were starting to miss out on days out. Every outing was starting to be a major plan.

"Yes, we can go there, they don't have Wi-Fi there - no we can't go there - there are mobile phone masts very close by or on the top of the building." This is how it was.

How could I live in a world of electricity if it was going to do this to me? I could not see any way out of this; it was just getting worse and worse. I wanted to end this misery. I picked myself up off the lounge floor and walked into the kitchen. As I passed our tiled wall, I kicked out at it! I had to. Now, I'm not an abusive person, far from it, but I just had to release the build-up of anger, frustration, negative *'energy'* and sadness that was flowing through me. I didn't cause any damage to the tiles thankfully, but I certainly had a good go at the wall that day!

At this point, I just had to ring my friend Lin, I was in dire straits. I needed to speak to someone who knew what I was going through, who knew my story. It wasn't right to ring Karl on this morning because he would have panicked and returned from work, I didn't want to worry him. I had met Lin through my music teaching. Both her boys received lessons from me. Lin had helped me so much up to now, she was a holistic healer and had kept me sane. When I made the telephone call, I was literally screaming and sobbing down the phone.

"I can't do this anymore! I just can't go on like this! I hate living like this! What's the point anymore?" I was inconsolable.

Lin tried her very best to console me, but it wasn't really working. I had got myself that worked up to a point where nothing was going to shake me out of it … nothing! I felt completely and utterly out of control. Finally, after a good amount of talking to, I eventually calmed down and came round. Lin remained calm throughout the whole conversation. I can't thank her enough for that day, for listening and understanding. She allowed me to feel the deep emotions that were running through me, not blocking it, letting it run free from me.

"Let it flow, allow the tears to flow, release those emotions, let it go."

Looking back, it was the right thing to do. There's nothing worse than trying to suppress negative feelings within you, they just seem to fire up even more, burning deeper inside you. The longer you hold onto them, the worse they get!

It was at this point she said, *"I think it's time to go and see Mike."*

Lin had mentioned Mike to me in the previous months. She had told me about hypnotherapy and hypnosis, saying how in a hypnosis session you can 'anchor' things to help you respond differently.

"Mike can anchor an action or a word whilst you are in hypnosis. You can then use it if you get symptoms. It may help. It may alleviate your symptom's."

I responded with *"That sounds really interesting. That would be amazing if I could do something like that!"*

Lin had previously told me about a quote with regards to creating 'beliefs', 'perceptions' and 'experiences'. It now made a lot of sense and resonated with me …

We create what we believe …
We believe what we perceive …
We perceive what we experience …
We experience what we create … *(anon)*[1]

This quote just keeps repeating itself over and over - it was about to make much more sense to me over the coming months.

I was clutching at straws, anything to escape this horrible feeling of not being free to live. I had previously read a Brian Weiss book called 'Many Lives, Many Masters'[2] which someone had kindly lent me, so I had a little understanding regarding hypnosis and past life regression, but I didn't really know that much about it at all at this point. I was now very desperate and open to any help I could get. I was lost in this world of being locked off from everyone and everything. Hypnotherapy sessions with Mike started the end of September and I instantly started to feel an escape route.

November 2007 saw the arrival of an acoustic piano at our house. All my keyboard instruments which I taught on had all been electric up until now. It was becoming painful to teach. I had to put things in place to help me - to be kind to me. I had to decide to help myself and ease the contact with electrical equipment for a period whilst on my healing journey. My diary shows this (Chapter 9). It helped tremendously. Sometimes we must take what seems to be a step back to move forward.

A Way Will Be Found

We all experience adversity at some point in our life. What we choose to do with that adversity can take us one way or the other. It can be life changing, either way, good or bad. We do have a choice in any 'moment'. Adversity and being in the depths of despair always seems the worst place you can be in that 'moment'. Sometimes you can't see the wood for the trees because you can't think straight, just like I experienced that morning after taking Ethan to school. I was out of control, completely! That morning my 'fight - flight - freeze' certainly appeared! Logical thinking disappeared and deep panic set it. I had nowhere to go, nowhere to hide. I was being threatened by something I couldn't even see!

When we are out of control, logic just disappears; shutting down the parts of our brain that allow us to flow and make decisions from a place of clear-headedness that will benefit us fully. This is known as our 'sympathetic nervous system'. The autonomic response known as FFF (Fight - Flight - Freeze) kicks in to protect us. It's our body's stress response when it perceives a threat, thinking we are in danger, causing psychological changes to deal with the situation at hand. During a stress response, our cortisol levels rise. Cortisol is often called the 'stress hormone', causing an increase in heart rate and blood pressure preparing you for the fight! I often nickname our 'fight - flight' response as our 'caveman syndrome'. It has kept us alive for thousands of years. We can't live without it. Imagine being faced with a sabre-toothed tiger all those years ago! Your 'sympathetic nervous system' response would have been on super overdrive only having a spear to defend yourself. All other thoughts go out the window and you respond accordingly to protect yourself. Another good example is a rabbit in the headlight's scenario. On the flip side, our 'parasympathetic nervous system' is our quiet, rest and digest response; it turns off the stress reaction. We are calm, relaxed, open to all options around us, because we can think clearly. There is no threat, conserving energy ready for use when we require it. The 'parasympathetic' creates the balance between the two responses, which we need to live a healthy life. Stress becomes a problem when we can't switch it off. It's almost like the 'sympathetic' response gets stuck. This comes from practised thought processes and responses that sink down into the subconscious part of our mind becoming a habit. Imagine the practised thought processes I was programming in continuously - adding to the 'fear' of electricity! You can see how something like that would develop over time. This could be related to any traumatic response in life.

If we can learn that our out-of-control feeling is just a 'moment', that it will pass, or change, we can start to refocus ourselves from that point quickly. Not allowing that feeling that's been creating unwanted beliefs, thoughts, responses and habits within us to take over us - we can start to shift our thoughts and trust a change will take place. Nothing is static, life is always changing and moving - just like our 'sympathetic' and 'parasympathetic' responses flow in and out in our daily life. It's how we develop and survive. All we require is a small trigger; that trigger could be the understanding above. Remembering 'choice' in any moment of where we focus. If we can find it deep within ourselves, even just a miniscule, we can start to move out of the adversity, using it as a guidance of redirection or reflection. Use the adversity to create the change. If I hadn't have got to that severe point in my life, I would have just kept plodding on trying to sort it out, probably going round in circles. That morning tipped me right over the edge and made me look for help, driving me to search and look in directions that I would not have considered had this not happened. So, is what happened a bad thing? No ... not necessarily; it became my driving force to find a way. Remember it's what we do with the adversity that makes all the difference. If we can see the adversity as that driving force to guide us, we can start to look at difficult situations in our life as blessings in disguise, trusting that that moment will pass. It must; we live in a continuously moving universe. After all, we only ever have NOW. Our subconscious mind only understands NOW. How we respond NOW determines our future and only ourselves can change that!

Hypnotherapy was about to change my life - change my thought processes and understandings of how I processed life. Hypnotherapy was about to save my life!

References:
[1] *We create what we believe.* Quote. (n.d.). (anon).

[2] Weiss, B. (1994). *Many Lives, Many Masters. Piatkus.*

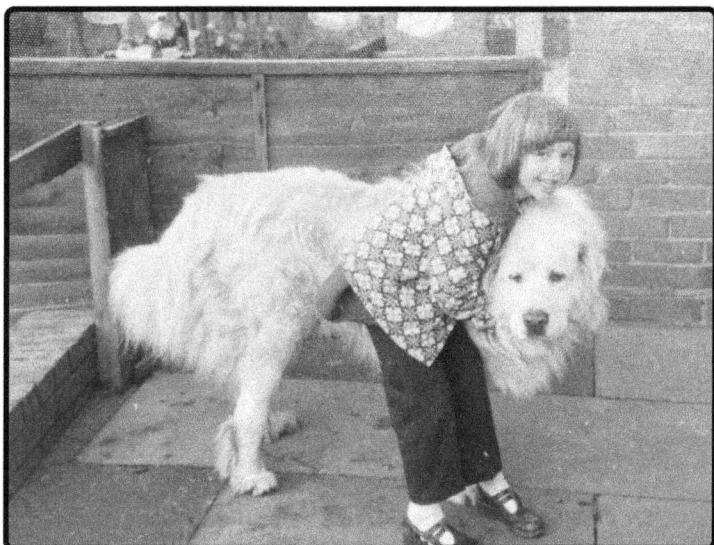

Me, with Snowy my Pyrenean Mountain Dog, c. 1976.

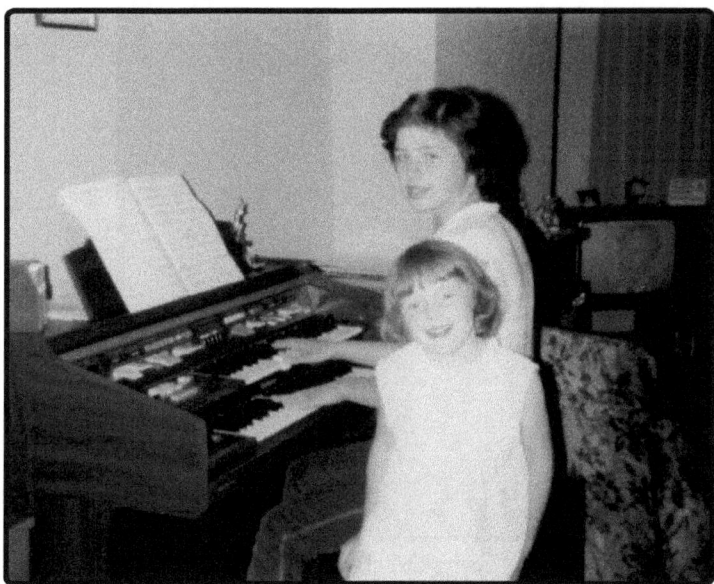

Playing electronic organ with my sister, Emma, c. 1985.

The mobile phone mast we walked up to
whilst in Chester, 2008.

During my course of chemotherapy treatment
- away in our caravan in Wales, April 2010.

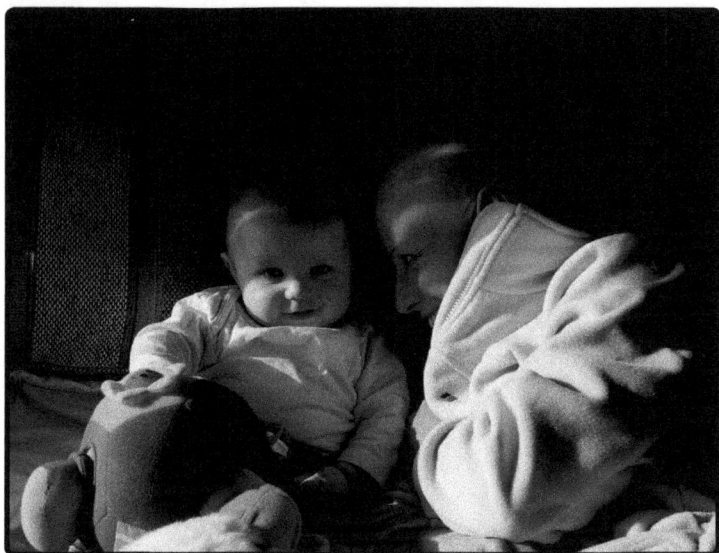

Me, with my nephew having a rest at our caravan, May 2010.

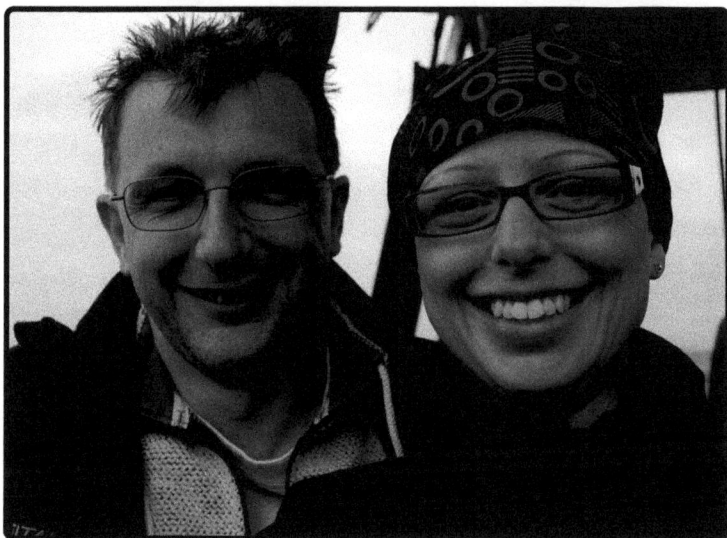

Our hot air balloon flight from Shugborough Hall Estate
on 23rd July 2010 - my last day of treatment.

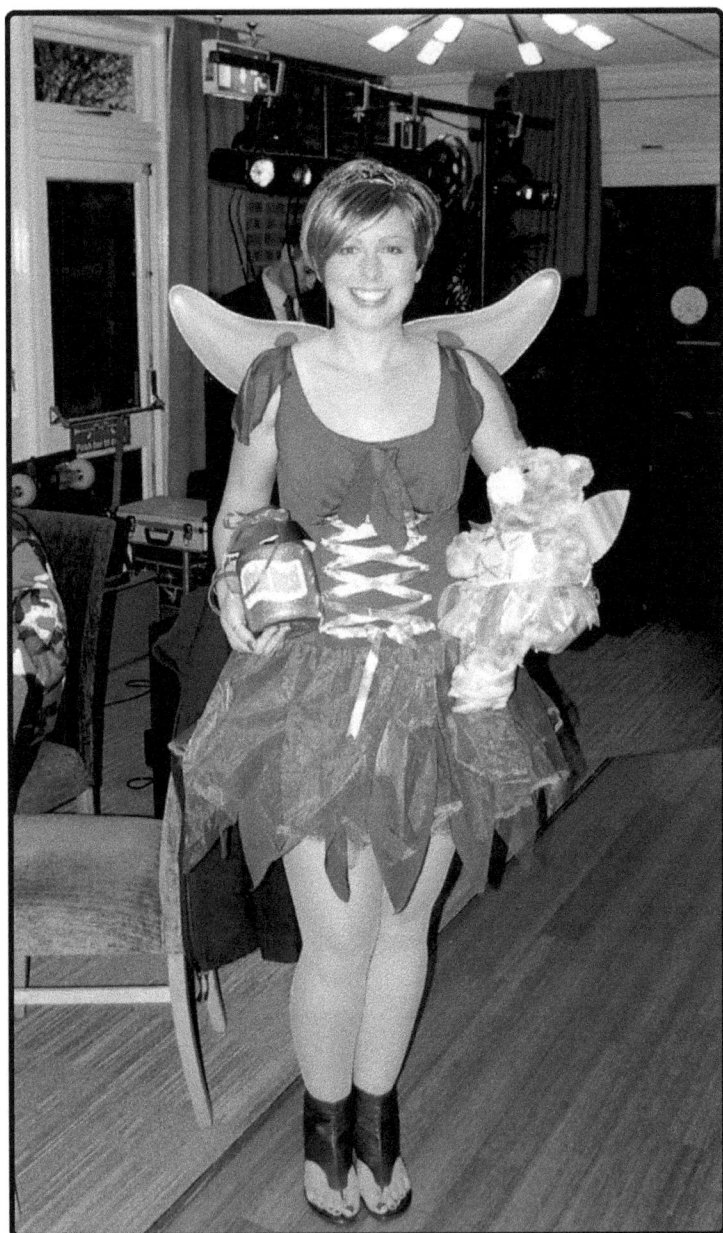

Dressed up as a fairy at my 40th birthday party,
September 2010.

Part II
Understanding the Mind

Michelle Townsend

Chapter 8

Hypnotherapy to the Rescue

'Fear comes in many forms ... face fear ... it adds to your wisdom. It's just the journey of life. Live it!'

'Paying attention NOW allows you to conduct this moment on purpose ...
just like a beautiful piece of music'.

~ Michelle Townsend

After that awful morning breaking down to my friend over the phone, I took on her advice to give hypnotherapy a go. Lin made the appointment for me. I was in dire straits, so I needed to find some way of relieving the symptoms. I couldn't go on any longer. There just had to be a way.

It was **Monday 1st October 2007**. Lin picked me up and took me to Mike's house for my 5.00pm appointment. We went in together, where she introduced me to Mike. I was in such a state, exhausted from everything that had been going on. Energy had left me, and my lack of interest in life was at an all-time low. I was feeling very insecure and vulnerable; I just felt so weak. Lin agreed to wait outside in the car for me.

Hypnotherapy was about to change my life forever. Change in the way I thought and change in the way I processed information from the reality around me, allowing a new way of thinking and living life. Mike explained about the subconscious part of our mind, and how hypnosis can help create positive change. I was amazed at what I was hearing. Having this understanding was allowing me to look at my responses in a completely different way. It was interesting and fascinating. But could this really help?

I share the first entry from my *'Dear Diary'* below. All other entries can be found in Chapter 9 - showing how things progressed over the time that I was having hypnotherapy sessions with Mike. When I read back through my diary entries, I can now identify, as a hypnotherapist myself, the different tools and techniques used by a therapist. It's extremely powerful stuff.

Monday 1st October 2007

Hypnosis session with Mike England - 5pm.

I really wasn't worked up about going for hypnosis because I was so desperate for this to work. I was exhausted, crying out for help. Mike explained everything to me. As he was guiding me into hypnosis, I could feel my heart pounding and my eyelids twitching. I kept thinking to myself ... *'Just relax. How will I know when I'm under?'* The thing is you don't! Mike guided me through a relaxation, telling me to think of a beach, flowers, the sky, sea, anything where I felt relaxed. I immediately went to Dunrobin Castle. A special place to me, a place where we have visited in Scotland. For some reason I felt safe there, relaxed. This was 'my safe place' for resting points through the hypnosis. Mike asked me to go back into the past, thinking of all the pictures I could remember and memories of my lifetime.

You work back and see many things you have done. He then asked if any of these were relevant, standing out more than others? I found myself in an electronics lesson when I was in senior school; it was only in the 1st year there. Our electronics teacher was showing us how to use oscillator machines which show frequency and how they are measured. Suddenly, I heard an extremely high-pitched sound in my ears; it was horrible. Although at the time it probably wasn't that bad, I didn't realise until this hypnotherapy session that I did put my hands to my ears, and ever since then my ears have been buzzing with tinnitus. Weird! It made me feel a bit funny. Had this registered a trauma in my body? Mike asked me how I felt as a young girl in that situation.

I replied ... *"It's like a shock to the system! I felt unhappy about it and didn't like it."*

He then told me to float above that situation as an adult and look at the young girl from that perspective.

He then asked ... *"How is the girl feeling now?"*

I replied ... *"She is associating the frequency to a musical note! It's ok!"*

Mike instructed me to let the young girl walk towards me and let her say how she feels now. *"She is smiling, she's happy, not bothered by the situation!"* ... was my response.

I may have left a few things out, but this is what I remember. I was then brought forward to now, and guided to see the changes made, visualizing the next 24 hours.

"See yourself driving your new car to the garage not affecting you, feeling happy. Just visualizing the next 48 hours."

Mike continued ... *"A lot happier, enjoying having fun again with your children. Now move on a week - just happier enjoying life not feeling trapped, just getting on with life. Moving into the next month - very happy driving your car, you can go where you want to, enjoying family life with no limitations."*

I was then told to imagine driving my car speeding around (not literally of course!), using my mobile phone in the centre of Birmingham (the city had just become a Wi-Fi city around this time), sending e-mails on the computer, free to do what I wanted to do. My arms when I came out of hypnosis had no pain in them at all. WOW! On the evening of my first hypnosis session, I felt great. Positive attitude, laughing and joking, rather than feeing exhausted. I felt such a relief!

It's at this point in my life that one book was about to open doors for me. That book was called 'The Secret'[1] by Rhonda Byrne. It's a beautifully presented book full of quotes from inspirational writers and speakers about the 'law of attraction'. It covers thoughts about things, the benefits of gratitude, beliefs, affirmations and the like. After reading Rhonda's book, I got engrossed in buying others from the authors that had appeared in it. I became aware of a couple who were supposed to be part of 'The Secret' book, but had decided to withdraw and write their own. This then led me onto the Esther and Jerry Hicks books starting with 'Ask and it is given.'[2] It was this book that really projected me into a 'vortex' as Esther would say, of how I could change my world around me. It all fitted in with the hypnotherapy sessions I was receiving. I became engulfed in this new way of thinking that was changing my life for the better. I couldn't believe it! Well, I could, because things were starting to change in my reality. I became fascinated by positive quotes about the mind and thoughts. I was about to find out how true Dr Wayne Dyer's words really were ...

'We become what we think about all day long.
The question is "What do you think about?" ' [3]

What had I been thinking all these years? Where had my mind been? I had been too focused on the reality in front of me and believing it to be true, creating more of the same.

We may question that reality is reality and we cannot change it. But we do have a certain amount of control over it by the thoughts that we think. It's only our perception of it. *'Thoughts have frequency'. 'Thoughts create things'*. How we think brings more of the same to us, and because we are focused that way, we create the belief that it is true. It cannot be any other way. What's true for one isn't necessarily true for another. So, what is true? This is how my thoughts about life were changing. According to Gandhi (n.d.)[4] ...

> *'Your beliefs become your thoughts,*
> *Your thoughts become your words,*
> *Your words become your actions,*
> *Your actions become your habits,*
> *Your habits become your values,*
> *Your values become your destiny'.*

The bizarre thing with all of this was I was married to an electrician! Thankfully, I wasn't allergic to my hubby! Karl understood electrical items gave off a frequency. There were times when we would walk into an electrical shop at our local shopping centre where he too would pick up the frequency from the lights. He agreed with me that they created a weird feeling. Even Karl experienced aches in his arms and a headache after he had been in there.

During the time I was attending hypnotherapy with Mike and building a recovery, we experimented with different situations and noted the effects from different electrical items. Most of them I knew about, but there were times when I didn't. Karl was intrigued to see if it was 'mind over matter'. Was I imagining it? He never doubted me, but felt he had to rule out my observations of this.

There were two specific times when Karl planned to test the 'mind over matter' scenario. Whilst I was teaching one evening, Karl installed Wi-Fi in our home. I was oblivious to what he was up to. After finishing work that evening, I sat down in the armchair in our lounge. I wasn't aware that Karl kept watching me to see if I would react or say something.

After about an hour I said ... *"Ooh, I feel funny."*

Karl responded ... *"In what way?"*

"I feel like I have been using my mobile phone," I replied.

"Right," he said. *"I haven't done this because I don't believe you, I've done it to see what happens. While you've been working, I have installed Wi-Fi in the house."*

At that, he instantly stood up and went to turn it off. It confirmed to him that I could pick up the frequency waves that the Wi-Fi was emitting. I wasn't angry, in fact I was relieved, because it proved it could happen. I wasn't going insane! Karl then uninstalled the technology and returned it to the shop, thankfully receiving a refund.

Another time Karl tested the waters, was whilst we were on holiday in Wales. We had the old truck at the time - a Mitsubishi Pajero for towing our caravan. I felt safe in this car; the electrics didn't affect me - well I believed they didn't. I was already aware we had the Sat-Nav in the car, but never used it because of the pain it caused me. One day, travelling to Llechwedd Slate mine near Ffestiniog, unbeknown to me, Karl had set the Sat-Nav for the trip but turned the volume down and hid it under the driver's seat.

Reaching our destination, he said ... *"You ok?"*

"Yes, why?" I replied.

"Well, you have just travelled all the way from the caravan to here with the Sat-Nav switched on and working; I've had it switched on under my seat."

I looked at him in surprise. *"Really?"*

"Yes!" he said.

"WOW!" ... was my response.

This wasn't a short journey we had just taken either. This was allowing my belief around the effects to change. We also visited the Dinorwig Power Station, otherwise known as 'Electric Mountain', near Dinorwig, Llanberis in Snowdonia National Park, North Wales. Even the name of the place created a panic in me, a feeling of dread, but I was determined we visited. I kept facing the fear, putting myself in situations deliberately so that I could put into practice what Mike had worked with during my hypnotherapy sessions. It became my project to find more and more electrical objects and situations to connect with, no longer backing away from it.

One caravan site we ventured to was near Delamere Forest, in Cheshire. We spotted a large mobile phone mast in the distance not too far away.

"I want to walk up to that mast." I said, one day during our holiday.

Karl, myself, and the boys then set out on a walk. I walked up as close as I could get to the mobile phone mast. I was so proud of myself. Each time I was placing myself in these situations it was creating a new belief, a belief that it was getting easier and easier, better and better. I kept on going. I believed I could do it! I finally connected to the belief that I could change my responses to the EMFs.

A Way Will Be Found

My hypnotherapy journey made me realise that it is so important to ask for help when we require it. Adversity can become a blessing when we accept where we are; it opens the door for change. Digging ourselves deeper into adversity only allows more of the same to flow into our lives. Having the awareness that change is possible can be the missing piece of the puzzle. Once that piece is in place, we can create the picture, unravelling the puzzle, creating new perceptions, allowing new beliefs to arise.

In my first few chapters of my book, I've touched upon and talked briefly about the conscious and subconscious mind, beliefs, perceptions and *'energy'*. Let us now develop a deeper understanding as we move further through my story, as to what I have come to understand by changing my perceptions. If we have just a simple understanding of how the mind works, we can start to move mountains that we never thought possible to move. Releasing deep seated emotions, responses from old experiences, fears, phobias and even illness. They are of course all 'energetic'. Our whole life works from a place of frequency. Thoughts have frequency. They have POWER!

Conscious and Subconscious Mind

We have two parts to our mind: our *'conscious mind'* and our *'subconscious mind'*. Liken it to a massive iceberg. The ice that floats above the water represents our conscious mind, which is analytical, making decisions and deals with the planning and verbalising ideas. It is the problem solving and reasoning part of our brain, working in numbers, is logical and sequential. It accounts for just 5% of our brain. The iceberg which lies beneath the water is always so much bigger. This represents our subconscious mind, holding so much more information. The subconscious is our emotional part, the part that deals with our feelings, emotions and memories. It carries out the decisions made by our conscious part, creating the interest, playing out programs and conditioning, it is the creative part of the mind. The subconscious runs our bodily functions, including our breathing, heartbeat, temperature, our autonomic systems, such as our fight - flight survival mechanism. It is also our habit centre, and my - does it love habit! Accounting for 95% mind power, the subconscious is definitely the BOSS!

Memories

We can't consciously remember and recall every experience we have had; we would be bombarded with way too much information. However, our subconscious remembers every millisecond of our life right the way back to the third trimester in our mother's womb. Imagine your subconscious like the folders on your computer. Each file holds certain memories and experiences that are similar. We have folders for happiness, holidays, achievements, successes etc. We also have folders for fear, sadness, phobias, unhappy times. As we experience life, the subconscious 'pattern matches' to our old experiences and places the memory in the relevant folder, adding to the information. It then uses the information stored to help us as we walk through life, bringing forward responses, beliefs and perceptions from what we have previously learnt. If an experience has strong emotions related to it, the subconscious takes it on board in a much more powerful way. This is great if we have positive experiences and learn new things that can project us further in life. However, if it starts to place memories of fear, phobias, negative experiences etc - and it will - into those relevant folders, it can start to create havoc. In turn, this creates limiting beliefs and thoughts associated with things of similar experience and can stop us moving forward. Afterall, our subconscious wants to protect us and its only way of doing that is from what it has picked up along the way on our life's journey - it has no other comparison. This is why people perceive life so differently. We all have different experiences and look at the same thing in a slightly different way.

The *'subconscious'*, otherwise known as the 'monkey brain' can play tricks on us, hence the 'monkey brain' title. Time does not exist in the subconscious mind; it only works with NOW! It does not distinguish between reality, or whether we are imagining/thinking it. It believes either to be true. This is why our thoughts have power in any moment.

Whatever thoughts we think right NOW, whether a past event, or projecting our thoughts into the future, worrying about a future event, our subconscious believes it to be happening right NOW! It doesn't distinguish past, present and future. The subconscious just takes our thoughts as truth, happening now and responds accordingly from the memories it holds about that subject. So, if thinking about a wonderful happy holiday memory, its likely feelings of happiness and excitement related to that will come forth. On the other hand, thoughts regarding a past event - that created fear or a traumatic response within - will likely bring forward feelings and responses that are uncomfortable. Anxiety and panic attacks can appear because the subconscious believes it must protect us from the current situations or experience. If, in a previous event the response was an anxious one, the subconscious pattern matches it, because this is how it has been taught to respond. It almost goes 'DING! alarm required'. This is just like that trauma from the year 2000. This is how we must now respond. Flick the switch - let's make Michelle respond this way! This is why we learn from our experiences.

It's important to understand these responses because we can then consciously start to change them, perceiving them from a different angle. Most people will say *'I **have** anxiety'.* We've all been there. We don't **have** anxiety. We **DO** anxiety. It's a choice. That's a hard one for people to assimilate and they will argue till they are blue in the face saying ... *'Yes. I **do have** anxiety. This is how I respond. I can't help it.'* These responses are coming from a subconscious level that has been practised consciously over time - that has sunk deep down, creating a belief leading to anxiety and responding that way. Anxiety comes from just one thing, 'a thought.' It can't come from anywhere else - it's our thoughts that trigger it - but it's good to know that thoughts can be changed.

It is commonplace for our subconscious to run at an automatic level without realising. We think this is how it should be and how our body works. If we chose to stop in any moment when experiencing something uncomfortable - being aware that we could change our perspective on that situation - and create a new model of programming to enter our subconscious - imagine what could change. Almost like consciously having a filter before we allow anything to enter deeper, penetrating the subconscious, which could then become a habit. I learned to use my conscious mind as the watchman at the gate. I became aware. Not allowing thoughts to sink down into my subconscious that had no benefit to me. I let those thoughts go. Dr Joseph Murphy tells us this in his amazing book 'The Power of your Subconscious Mind'[5] (2008). It is Dr Murphy's book that became my bible. It was a life changer. As I consciously started to change my thoughts and understanding they were just a 'thought' - the responses changed. It's the same with most things. I learned I was only one thought away from feeling calm, one thought away from feeling relaxed. Acknowledging my thoughts in that moment and consciously changing that thought response was key. My subconscious then started to respond accordingly, taking on the information, logging it away. This is what I was doing with EHS. I was changing the program. Liken this to updating an 'app' on a phone or computer - we do updates to sort out the bug fixes. If we can sort **our** bug fixes out by changing our thoughts, our subconscious 'app' will then update. This also relates to 'neuroplasticity', but more on this later. Remember the saying, 'if you don't use it, you lose it!' I started to use and keep the thoughts I wanted. This was the start of a new way of life for me.

'Whatever we plant in our subconscious mind and nourish with repetition and emotion will one day become our reality.'[6]

~ Earl Nightingale

'Thoughts become things. If you see it in your mind, you will hold it in your hand.'[7]

~ Bob Proctor

Most of our life is on autopilot running at a subconscious level. We spend most of our life in hypnosis. For example, we don't think about how we do certain tasks, such as how we get up in a morning, how we make our first drink, how we drive to work. We just do it, usually consciously thinking about something completely different whilst in the process. Ever driven somewhere and have no idea how you got there? We learn and it becomes automatic. From this understanding I knew that my responses had to change, it was obvious they would. Why wouldn't they? Proof was starting to appear in front of me.

Be aware of this subtle understanding when reading my dear diary entries. It's food for thought. Connecting into new possibilities.

'Our greatest glory is not in never failing, but in rising up every time we fail.'[8]

~ Ralph Waldo Emerson

References:

[1] Byrne, R. (2000). *The Secret.* Simon & Schuster Ltd.

[2] Hicks, E. and Hicks, J. (2004). *Ask and It Is Given: Learning to Manifest Your Desires.* Carlsbad: Hay House.

[3] Dyer, W. (2004). *The Power of Intention.* Hay House.

[4] Gandhi, M. (n.d.). *Your beliefs become your thoughts.* [Online] Available : https://www.goodreads.com/ quotes/50584-your-beliefs-become-your-thoughts-your-thoughts-become-your-words

[5] Murphy, J. (2000). *The Power of your Subconscious Mind.* London. Pocket Books.

[6] Nightingale, E. (1956). *The Strangest Secret.* [Online] Available at: https://www.goodreads.com /quotes/218390-whatever-we-plant-in-our-subconscious-mind-and-nourish-with

[7] Proctor, B. (1997). *You Were Born Rich.* Life Success Productions.

[8] Emerson, R.W. (1841). *Self-Reliance.* James Munroe and Company, Boston.

Michelle Townsend

Chapter 9

Dear Diary

'It is what it is ... use it as guidance'.

~ Michelle Townsend

From **October 2007**, when my symptoms got exceedingly worse, I felt it necessary to keep a diary of my progress following my first hypnotherapy session. I have included what I feel is relevant to give a full understanding of my experience and what I was going through. The diary section is as it was written. Nothing has been edited here. It's warts and all! You will see how my thought processes were working at that time, how negatively focused I had become, how I had programmed myself.

Doing the simplest of daily things became a major task. *'Dear Diary'* gives a glimpse of this short space of time - how EHS affected me and how I improved. How I maintained my focus, but also how I felt like giving up! Certain entries may seem silly to some, but it was very real for me. My words highlight where my *'energy'* was at this time; showing the sheer desperation to be freed from the intense pain I was experiencing. Compared with how I have written most of my book, the shift can be clearly seen, not only in *'energy'* and my thoughts, but in my feelings and responses. A complete turnaround. Each entry is written in note form - my aim being to write down how I was feeling at that time.

These diary entries continue from the day after my first hypnotherapy session, which I have shared in Chapter 8. This was my life.

Tuesday 2nd October 2007

Woke feeling good, just a little achy. Drove the car to school and it reminded me of driving my Mini Cooper - relaxing and fun. I got back home and arms were burning a little. I didn't let it sway me though. Drove the car back to the garage as some paint work needed correcting on it. I mean - a new car!!! We were to be without it for about 10 days. It started affecting my arms on the way. Great ... I thought! But never mind; my cells have got to adjust; I just need time. What I had noticed today was that it wasn't zapping my energy levels, they remained high. By the evening, when I was working my arms were burning and in pain, my shoulders had gone tense. I took a paracetamol, and it eased it. Energy levels remained high though. Went to bed comfortable.

Wednesday 3rd October 2007

Woke feeling sorry for myself. Had a cry and cleared it out my system and took control again. I still had loads of energy it wasn't lapsing. I spoke to my healer, Lin, and she reassured me. We did another Bach Remedy to help with the emotions. Mike contacted me and was pleased my energy had remained high. He told me to start introducing things back into my life as each day passed - the computer, mobile phone etc. I asked if there was anything I could say to myself to help maintain positivity. He suggested - *'I am leaving the old condition behind, moving to a new feeling of freedom and perfect health.'* With this statement I would think of when Mike told me to look in the mirror at the new me! New body! Step into the mirror and watch the old body crumble away. Also think of that young girl smiling now. For pain relief, I need to tell my body *'Ok, you're telling me there's a problem - just let it go now the issue is being resolved.'* Later that evening, after being in contact with electrical items, the pain remained, but I stayed positive. I overcame it emotionally by saying the affirmations to myself. The good thing was I didn't take any paracetamol that evening and still my energy levels were on a high. It didn't knock me down. I had done so much more than I usually physically coped with that day. Moving forward. Moving forward. Yippee!

Thursday 4ᵗʰ October 2007

Decided to rest today and relax. Working with affirmations.

Friday 5ᵗʰ October 2007

Spent a couple of hours on my computer today to catch up with work. I did fine, a few sensations but it was more like a cooling feeling, I noticed there was no loss of co-ordination or energy. I worked that evening and later went to rehearsals for the church band, a few sensations but overall, not really a problem. Good. Good. Good!

***

During this time, I was helping some friends with their church band playing keyboard. I'm not a church goer, as my beliefs come from a place of seeing God as *'energy'*, everything around us. I thoroughly enjoyed my time with them. It also helped me to work with the sensations I was experiencing with my keyboard. Putting me in positions to overcome it.

***

Saturday 6ᵗʰ October 2007

Had a little trouble focusing today but got through it. Performing at church this evening. During performance, I got a little frustrated with chord sequence, then suddenly, I felt as though the electronics were affecting me. I was surrounded by electrical wires and equipment. *'Oh no,'* I thought *'not now'* and panicked inwardly. I could have cried, but I remembered what Mike had told me ... *'when you feel pain, or it is affecting you, say to yourself ... It's ok, I know there's a problem, let it go, the problem is being resolved.'* Eventually it worked, it bought me back into balance. I then had a sudden surge of confidence, and I just went into full flow on stage, improvising. I was really enjoying myself. I had some lovely compliments on my playing - it made my day. Thank you!

Sunday 7ᵗʰ October 2007

Tense today, kept trying to relax but sensations didn't ease. We decided to go out for lunch and I switched off from it all. Raided the shopping centre and hubby treated me to cheer me up. Once home, we watched TV (which I was ok with at this time). It was all I was capable of but looking forward to my session with Mike again tomorrow.

Monday 8ᵗʰ October 2007

Hypnotherapy session today, second session with Mike. He asked me how I'd been getting on. I told him that it wasn't affecting my energy levels anymore, but had been suffering with my arms. I told him the affirmations had been working well.

I was taken into hypnosis again where Mike asked me... *"Is there anything or a place we needed to go to resolve this issue?"*

My subconscious mind said ... *"Unsure, didn't know, no not really."*

He then directed me onto thinking about all these things that were affecting me. Mobile phones, masts, computer, car, electronics etc and worked on all the frequency waves.

He then said ... *"Imagine all the waves entering my body and throwing a party because they are getting on with my body, organs, blood, cells, everything a 'celebration'."*

Mike placed his hand on my right hand and said ... *"Imagine there is a balloon attached to your middle finger, but it is black and dark. Put all the things in there that you want to be rid of, things that you don't want to experience anymore and imagine the balloon getting bigger, filling it with these things."*

Mike then placed his hand on my left hand and said... *"Imagine this as a beautiful, coloured balloon. Fill this balloon with everything you want to improve. Good, fantastic feelings, driving your car, using the computer, playing keyboard, using a mobile phone etc but most of all, to be there for your family and to be able to do everything you want to do with your husband and children; no limitations to where you can go."*

Mike then asked me to release the black right-hand balloon into the atmosphere and let it go for good. It went up into space. The balloon in the left hand he told me to keep it, and place it somewhere in my body; so, I placed it right by where I had been told about some tissue mass by my thymus gland, and there it lives sorting out the issues. I came out of hypnosis feeling very tired, but was relaxed and fine. I was advised that if the pain appears again, to imagine a river and say no to the pain, 'laugh at it', let it run away down river. 'GOODBYE!' - not having this anymore! I'm going to enjoy myself (River Analogy). My confidence is getting better now, I can deal with people better. My new affirmation *'My body is becoming more and more comfortable accepting all frequencies with freedom from pain.'*

Tuesday 9ᵗʰ October 2007

Woke with stomach cramps. Felt like I had tummy bug. Karl borrowed an ELF (Extremely Low Frequency) monitor to try against electrical equipment. Green light meant low field, yellow light meant moderate fields and red light meant warning of high field. He said his dad's car was showing nothing! Our new car was fluctuating around yellow. We put it by the computer. It was really low and stayed green. We went round the house and by the wires, light switches, lights and television; they were all reaching red. My keyboard and piano shockingly enough were on full warning, high field; get your head round that one! We even tried a mobile phone; this remained on low until you started to ring a number, then it pulsed to maximum red! That evening, the computer, piano and keyboard were on. I felt the frequency from them, which I had been feeling for a few weeks, but had been dismissing it, which I will continue to do so! I must keep thinking positive as I write this now, I still have energy and my arms are not so bad. I have told it to ... *'go away, not accepting this anymore, it's past a joke ... be done with you!'* ... and it's helping. Although I took paracetamol about 3pm, they would have worn off now, so arms can't be too bad tonight after all.

Wednesday 10th October 2007

Woke up quite well today. Arms not really hurting too much. Had to do some work on the computer, so sat back from it and to the side, as I can still feel it. Kept telling myself to let the feelings go as the issue is being resolved and working with the river analogy. I had a small go on the piano to practise some aural tests and felt sensations in my arms, so took some paracetamol to help, as I was working tonight - 4pm till 9pm. I managed ok, although arms have suffered a bit tonight. By the time 8pm came, my arms seemed more settled and I felt relaxed. Again, I have noticed my energy is still good. Chest feels tight and pain in arms kept coming and going. Had a few heart palpitations, but feel really relaxed. Keeping positive thoughts; maybe this is what I need to go through to get through this!

Thursday 11ᵗʰ October 2007

Excited that we finally have the car back today. I prepared myself to accept that I probably would have some effect from it; this actually kept me positive because it wouldn't give me the negativity and upset like the last time. Again, it's accepting that there's a problem but let it go, the issue is being resolved. This has kept me positive all day. Mentally, I feel good and positive, but physically I am still very much reacting at the moment, today especially. I continued to focus positively, struggling through the pain in my arms and the feeling in my chest is back. My lymph nodes around my neck are feeling swollen as well. Co-ordination off, funny eyes and head today. Rang Lin to explain what's been happening and she reassured me and did some healing over the phone.

Over the time of all of this, I have suddenly noticed that I am working with the *'Phytobiophysics'*[1] essences 'Lightening Tree' and 'New Wave'. Because of my chest today, I have taken to 'Breathe' essence again and this has helped, along with the *'Bach Flower Remedies'*[2]. Used the car again and still felt some effect from it. It seems to put pressure on my chest and throat; my sensations are weird! Later returned home and felt better, arms not so painful - the effects seem to be wearing off better than before, although I do feel as though my head, chest and throat are still there slightly, but am telling it I'm dismissing it to 'let it go!'

***

The *'Phytobiophysics essences'* work on the principal that there is an invisible *'energy'* flow through the meridians of the body. It uses flower formulas which act as 'energy harmonisers' to bring the body back to a state of balance. Everything has a vibration, including disease. Disease can interfere with the body's *'energy'* flow, causing blockages, thus creating illness. Phytobiophysics helps to alleviate and stabilise the body's physical and emotional functions.

The *'Bach Flower Remedies'* are essences derived from flowers and plants. Each corresponds to a specific emotion, helping bring a sense of peace, balancing your emotions. Around this time, I received training from Lin on 'Bach Flower Remedies'.

You can see why I was working with Phytobiophysics and Bach Remedies because of their links with frequency to help balance my *'energy'* and emotions back then.

***

Friday 12th October 2007

Awoke quite refreshed today. Arms felt a little funny, achy, but ok. Karl asked me if I wanted the new car today and I said either way I don't mind, so I had the car. Took the boys to school and wasn't too bad at all. Later drove to Lin's, keeping positive all the time and it wasn't that bad. Got there and Lin had to take her son to school, so went with them in her car which I was ok with. Lin's car is new as well. When we got back, I needed to post a letter, so Lin came with me in my car to see how I reacted. I was ok.

I went into Lin's for some healing, and she channelled through from the guides. I can't remember a lot of it, but it was mentioned that the issue is a 'power' thing. In a previous life, I was a powerful person, and the pain is to do with being held back. The guides mentioned 'strength through playing' or 'playing with strength' is important; this is my music. She also mentioned when I realised the mobile phone was hurting my head, I was picking up negatives from the conversation and had associated with this; it then manifested. The healing went well; I was also sitting there before the healing session controlling the pain and reactions. Lin picked up that the pain in my arms is where someone has physically held me back and said 'no' and stopped me doing things. She mentioned the note C# in music, and said the note is relevant; also, the number 13. Whether this is to do with leading note resolving (that's a musical term by the way. Leading note is the note that appears before a return to the main keynote, the Tonic). She told me to work with the resonance of C# with my body and how it reacts. Designing clothes keeps coming up, and that I need to be practical with my hands, which in fact I am a very practical person and very good at sewing. As a child I used to make my own dolls' clothes, using my mother's sewing machine. I keep taking 'New Wave Essence' when I feel shaky and it's helping.

When I drove back, I didn't really feel any reactions from the car … WOW! So, I went to visit a friend and felt fantastic about it all, the best I have felt in two weeks. My friend asked me to check something on her keyboard and I picked up a little from this but drove the car fine to school. Worked tonight and wasn't too bad, quite full of life. Did rehearsal at the church late evening and only picked up small amounts from the piano. So, a really good day today.

Saturday 13th October 2007

Woke up feeling awful, tired and no motivation at all. Worked today music teaching and luckily had two theory and two practical, so wasn't on the keyboard or piano much. I needed to do some sounds for the church performance that was taking place that evening because it was the 'Harvest' service, but really couldn't get motivated. Went to church with a headache and aches. Feeling a bit off balance but enjoyed the night. Still tired. Paracetamol helped.

Sunday 14th October 2007

Didn't get up until 12.20pm today and again I am so, so tired, feeling off balance and generally funny/horrible - just want to sleep. Spent most of the day nodding off. I really can't be bothered today. Although, as I write this, I have picked up a bit now but my arms, head and chest aches - I feel quite emotional. Oh well - tomorrow is another day.

Monday 15th October 2007

Feeling a little tired today. Driven car to school and picked up frequencies a little, but coped fine. Decided to work with the 'New Wave Essence', 'Bach Remedies' and positive thinking today. Fetched children from school, but started to pick up frequencies from car, so wasn't in a very good mood when Karl returned from fishing. Karl said we'd take the truck (our older car) to take the children swimming, but I said ... *'no - we will go in the new car'*, and boy, was I picking up the frequencies! I remained calm and was fighting it off. Coped at swimming well and when we got home, I relaxed in the chair and pain eased. It felt like I controlled it tonight, although it is wearing me out. Try again tomorrow.

Tuesday 16th October 2007

Woke up tired again and eyes were burning and feeling a little raw and tender. Drove to school, but started to get twinges in my head, which made me feel like I was going to blackout at the wheel. At this point, I really felt I needed to have a rest from the car. I texted Karl to bring the truck back, so he could have the new one (Ford Focus ST) which he did. I rang Mike and he's going to get back to me (had to leave a message). Also rang Lin. She gave me some healing on my head over the phone which helped and made me feel positive again because I felt bloody awful, wobbly, co-ordination all over the place, sore eyes, achy arms, neck, shoulders, chest - whatever!!! Struggled on through the day and eased off gradually. Just my eyes mainly now. Arms start a little if on computer or keyboard/piano, but managing there. Took 'Lightening Tree Essence' with 'Bach remedies' today to help emotions.

Wednesday 17th October 2007

Awoke not too bad at all, just sore eyes. I really feel like I need lots of company at the moment, I get really fed up with the day and can't get motivated. Mom and Dad popped over today just to break it a little. Tried computer again for a short while but sat back from it. Fetched boys and teaching went well. Spoke to Mike quickly and this gave me positive thoughts and feedback. A good evening overall, feeling good but eyes just a little sore.

Thursday 18th October 2007

Feeling ok this morning. Ventured down to school in the truck and spoke to one of my friends. She asked me if I had seen the newsletter from HAS (Home and School Association) which I hadn't had time to read the night before. She informed me they are buying 16 wireless laptops for the school. At this I decided to go straight into school and speak to the head teacher about it raising my views on wireless technology, informing her of my illness and sensitivity. She did listen but couldn't promise they wouldn't buy them. I said I'd put a letter together and mention websites to look at. The rest of the day seemed to go much the same, but I kept busy and seemed to have good energy levels today. Felt a little washed out taking my eldest son swimming tonight and didn't really want to go on computer when I came back, but spent two and a half hours doing the letter for school. I had to sit back from the computer and managed ok.

Friday 19th October 2007

Lethargic today. Very tired this morning and my eyes are so sore and dry, hurting and runny. Headache pending as well - it did develop and had to take paracetamol to help. Having problems eating again today. There have been days where I really don't want anything to eat. I only had breakfast this morning and didn't have anything, only a chocolate just before I fetched my boys from school. I'm definitely grazing at the moment (eating when I feel I need to). Overall, a good day. Feel a bit shaky, but feel focused. Another session with Mike tomorrow. Keep positive we can do this!

Saturday 20th October 2007

Looking forward to my hypnosis session with Mike today. I had mentioned about 'regression therapy' to Mike previously. He said he would give me the option to 'regress' during hypnosis. If it was relevant and I needed to go to another place, then that would be the right time to go, but it's not always.

I explained that all I could concentrate on at the start of hypnosis was my heart going two to the dozen, so he went through a technique to help me through that and bring my heart rate down. Once in hypnosis, he told me to imagine a calm safe place. Mike spoke about when the EHS (Electromagnetic Hypersensitivity) started, asking where was my first recollection of pain from the mobile phone?

I said ... *"It was talking to a friend on the mobile, but it was plugged into the mains socket because my battery was flat, and I was talking for quite a while on it."*

He told me to imagine a mist and wanted me to walk through it ... *"I want you to look down at your feet. What are you wearing on your feet?"*

I wasn't sure to start with; all I could see was the mist. As I did walk through the mist, I thought I could see posh sandals with gold and jewels on the leather, which came up and wrapped round my calves.

"Scan around the area, float above the ground to see where you are."

I thought I said I was in Egypt as I saw the Pyramids, then I saw what I imagine looked like sugar beet with an alley running down the middle where there was a little mud hut. I was a young girl standing alone in the alley way between the sugar beet (do they have sugar beet in Egypt?) I was dressed in very posh clothes, a leather pleated mini skirt with jewels and gold around my neck. I had long jet-black hair, beautiful hair if I say so myself. A very beautiful young woman - but she was standing alone, no one about, completely alone.

Mike asked me ... *"What is going on around you? Move on to see what's happening."*

But I was just standing there, couldn't move. By this time, I was shaking in the hypnotherapy seat and felt cold and frightened.

Mike asked again and said ... *"It's ok. Why is she there?"*

I said ... *"I think she has been taken out there and abandoned because people don't like her views or what she is doing. She has done really well for herself, but people are jealous and envious and want to stop her."*

He then asked me ... *"Why do you think this is relevant to your present life?"*

I said ... *"I feel as though I have never been allowed my point of view, especially as a child. I do now, but while I was growing up, I felt I was held back and not allowed to do things I wanted to do, never allowed an opinion."*

He then took me back and said about things I wanted to keep and things I want to throw back into the mist.

"Imagine a backpack and you are keeping the good things but throwing the bad stuff back through the mist," which I did.

He then asked me ... *"How does that girl feel now? How does she feel while talking on the mobile phone in this life?"*

I said ... *"Much happier, not hanging onto other people's issues, just empathize with them."*

I can't really remember much more; I know we did talk about other things, but I can only really remember what I wrote.

Mike brought me out of hypnosis and we discussed the communication issue. In the regression, the issue was a girl being left, not being able to communicate. What is the EHS stopping me doing? 'Communicating!' I have always had issues about speaking to people and communicating. I always back off from confrontations and don't think I'm good enough to do things; very low esteem. Mike said I had to register this and link it together. He told me to think of this as all the past tense now. It's a little difficult when you're in pain and feeling shit from picking up frequencies. It's difficult staying positive all the time. I do try, but sometimes feel panicky, like there is no relief from it. I require to not focus on it and change my belief! Mike gave me a CD to listen to, for when I go to bed, just before I go to sleep to take away the negative thoughts and thought patterns (new beliefs need to be in place!) Going on holiday tomorrow, so ready to switch off for a while.

Sunday 21st October 2007

A good day travelling and lovely caravan site - nice and peaceful. Bought me a new book to read - Richard Hammond's autobiography.

Monday 22nd October 2007

Day trip to Wookey Hole today; really enjoyed it. It was very interesting, trying not to keep thinking about the last few weeks, but it's hard. Keep thinking about the school Wi-Fi - could do without this now. I am playing my CD every night and sometimes I fall asleep before it's finished.

Tuesday 23rd October 2007

Visited Bath today. We had a lovely walk round the town. Feel a bit out of it today - a little overwhelmed, as in some shops, the frequencies made my arms feel funny and my head woolly, but I shut it out and fought back.

Wednesday 24th October 2007

Stayed in our caravan today. Karl's mom and dad came down with their friends. We just had a relaxing day today, walked round the site and enjoyed the countryside.

Thursday 25th October 2007

Had a ride out to Cheddar Gorge. We didn't visit caves, but walked round the shops etc. We had a lovely dinner in the gorge, raided the cheese shop and had cheese and crackers! A quick drive to Weston-Super-Mare, Breen and Burnham. We just passed through them really. Visited Clarks Village Outlet, which is a retail park. A good day, but picked up stuff in the shops again, which I discarded. For some reason, I woke up in the night that evening, with my arms really hurting. Maybe it was because I was woken up, startled by Karl's mobile phone, after I had played my CD from Mike. I wasn't best pleased and couldn't really get back to sleep. Restless night. Paracetamol for headache today.

Friday 26th October 2007

I feel like being quiet today, but I had some good news. Karl informed me that there was Wi-Fi on the camp site. He had kept it from me deliberately, to see if I reacted. Karl hadn't realised when he had booked it that there was Wi-Fi on the site and apparently when we arrived on Monday, he mentioned to the reception about my illness - EHS.

The man was more than happy to turn it off, but Karl said to him ... *"No, it's not a problem. Could you leave it on, I want to see how my wife reacts without her knowing it's here. I will come back to you if we have any problems."*

Karl apologised for being so cruel to me, but said he wanted to prove something, which he did - I thank him for that. 'Mind over matter!' We stopped off at services on the way back and there was Wi-Fi in there. As we sat and had lunch, I noticed a man working on his laptop, who was probably on the Wi-Fi connection. I stayed calm and positive. I was picking it up, but brushed it off, reaping the effects later though! Played CD again and it relaxed me for a good night's sleep.

Saturday 27th October 2007

Enjoyed teaching today. Arms were very good when I started, but picked up piano and keyboard a little and threw me off balance. Took paracetamol to help and it eased the pain and sensations.

Sunday 28th October through to Sunday 11th November 2007

Yes, I've got to the stage where I don't want to write in my diary every day, but it's been a funny old two weeks! I'll give you an overall summary. An average of good and bad days, very emotional. Taking more time for family is special. I made the decision on the spur of the moment to buy an acoustic piano, due to the electronic instruments. Feel the need to do this very strongly, to allow me to recover and limit my contact with it. Need space. Hadn't realised it was time of the month

3rd November and on Friday 2nd November, felt poorly on the morning with my eye and head. Started to panic when I started my period; wondered why it was only 3 weeks? But it was 4 after all. Shows where my head is and what I'm concentrating on. Need to focus on things more. My piano came Monday 5th and has helped extremely throughout the week.

Saw Lin on Tuesday 6th. Had healing and has raised my *'energy'*. Had reassuring fairy cards this week - 'Positive Expectations' and 'Happy Ever After'. These have helped. Got all my newsletters and London College of Music work done. Getting myself up to date with everything. I personally think I've done well, considering what I'm having to cope with. I feel like people are ignoring me or avoiding me at the moment. They don't know how to deal with me or approach me. Maybe it's me imagining it. Am I really bothered NOT! Which is unusual for me - it's not me to be like that. Left to my own devices as usual! I'm only focusing on positive things now. I don't even bother with negatives if I can help it. Who needs them!

Lin is sending me healing every day, I must write down 1 - 10 on how I feel.

Sunday 11th November 2007

Slept all day. That's it really!

Monday 12th November 2007

Good day today. Appointment with Mike at 1pm. Mike explained he was going to show me how to do 'self-hypnosis' today and we will be working with the body itself, rather than emotional and mental issues. He explained he would turn music off during parts of the hypnosis this time. He asked if the CD had helped, which it has - wonderfully! I certainly know how to relax now and switch off. He took me into hypnosis, and I relaxed straight away, much easier than last time.

I can't remember much of the first part, but I remember Mike saying ... *"Float above yourself and look down at your body. Look what is happening."*

He asked me to see my body next to me, around 9 years ago, when I was well, before the problems started. He then told me to tune into my eyes and imagine the frequency they are resonating at and imagine it as a note in my head, then compare it with the body 9 years ago and see the difference, then to re-tune into the original frequency.

He asked ... *"Can you feel a change in your eyes? You will know when it's in place."*

We then worked with the kidneys, arms, legs, joints, heart and brain. Mike left me for about 10 minutes to do this myself. He was watching me but didn't speak. He then asked me to see if the whole orchestra was in tune, the conductor was conducting and what sound or music I could hear.

He told me ... *"Keep referring to the conductor to tune in and keep check."*

Mike at one point trained me to hypnotise myself. He held my hands in a position and said *"Relax, relax, relax"* ... by saying these words, it would put me into hypnosis - re-tuning my organs and parts of my body and check the conductor is doing his job. To finish the hypnosis, Mike took me through the next few weeks. He also asked me for a number. I said *"9"* straight away. This is the number of days I must do this 'self-hypnosis' retuning 'FREEDOM'. Once I had come out of the hypnosis, he went through the technique he had shown me and practised it. We talked about it and even suggested trying to find the notes on the piano for the different parts of my body and writing a song or playing them to maintain the resonance. Maybe this is why I desperately needed an acoustic piano? I need natural resonance for healing. Felt good this evening, but during the night, I awoke with very painful calves. Haven't had that for years. Maybe it's the healing process? A good day today!

Tuesday 13ᵗʰ November 2007

Positives today once I got going. Tidied up, hoovered, went on computer, which didn't affect me as much. Wasn't reacting against keyboard as much. These are good positives. Not sure what to think of 'self-hypnosis'. Hope I've done it right. Felt good tonight when I finished work.

Unsure of date - sometime in December 2007

Hello Diary, it's been a while. Sorry I've not been in touch for a month, but I've been working hard and assessing life!

Let me just analyse the past four weeks after the last session with Mike on Monday 12ᵗʰ November. I decided to ring him on the Thursday to reassure me of the 'self-hypnosis' process. I had been doing it slightly wrong and he reassured me what to do. Focusing on the past body and present future body and tune each organ and part of the body to remember when it was healthy etc. Funnily enough, all this stuff to do with retuning was linked with me having my acoustic piano, and it was resonating badly on the note B for some reason! I decided to continue tuning in my head and not work with the piano after the 9 days of doing it properly. I just kept on with the 'self-hypnosis', doing it on the overall body. Mike asked me to contact him after 10 days. I rang him and left a message, but his phone wasn't working right. A week later I tried again, but in the meantime, I carried on. Things had been positive. I very rarely look at things negatively at this stage, but on Karl's' moms' birthday we went over to take her present and his dad put a video on about the cruise. I started to feel myself getting upset, feeling I wouldn't be able to do that, go on a cruise, so I rushed upstairs and really cried.

Karl came up to me and snapped … *"You're being negative again!"*

This really upset me. After this, I cried all day for 13 hours or so. I even woke up on the Monday morning feeling tearful. It seemed, looking back now, an emotional release. Lin had mentioned 'release' as 'real-ease' from that day. I've not looked back and don't look at anything in a negative way whatsoever. I change it to the positive. I have noticed that my reaction to the instruments has diminished, and I can sit in front of the computer again now. There are daily fluctuations, but I still don't look at this negatively. For example - I helped Karl put our Christmas tree up and he asked me to hold the fairy lights, which had fibreoptics. It was switched on, and as I put my hand on it, the burning and tingling sensation I got was quite strong. I didn't back off and addressed it with ... *'I know you're there but let it go.'* I have also been using the ... *'It never affected me before, so why should it now?'* This strengthens me. I feel waves of positiveness wash over me. It's fantastic when I get this! When I did speak to Mike, he praised me up and said I have done fantastically! I explained that I was starting to get bored with the current 'self-hypnosis' and he told me to change it slightly and say the affirmation ... *'It's just so easy to move towards that future body where I am completely healthy, happy and confident - I am noticing improvements in my health every single day!'* I then worked with that in 'self-hypnosis', comparing the past body and remembering the feelings when I was well.

Mike also told me to 'self-hypnotise' before and after driving the car, to take it round the block on short drives and build up gradually. That has now improved. I really don't feel negative now. I can feel the changes.

Most of the time, I'm good physically, and when I do have a reaction, I just reassure myself and say ... *'You know I reacted before, but this time I'm going to be fine and see improvements.'* Lin suggested I go to get another blood test to check my B12, Folic Acid etc, because of the occasional fatigue. The doctor wasn't really that understanding when I went up! Got the bloods done and they have come back brilliant! Everything is within normal levels. The doctor was more understanding this time, but he said he didn't know what else he could do. He didn't know where to recommend me. He praised me up for doing the hypnosis sessions and to carry on what I was doing because I seem to have it under control. To go back if I need anything else, which was good.

My next session with Mike was just a chat and guidance how to carry on positively. He gave me a new affirmation to say just before my 'self-hypnosis' to do 10 minutes twice a day.

'My health has improved so much that my body remains completely healthy in all situations with all the items of electricity, Wi-Fi and other related items. I notice the effect of this healthiness immediately.'

He told me when I'm teaching on the electronic keyboard and organ to reinforce the word *'healthiness'.* If I react, get firm with it, tell it to go away and get out sternly.

I also need to be aware of how I feel every half hour/hour, change it with the above affirmation, and do this for 5 days - enough to saturate.

It's important now that I don't talk about it - even if feeling it. Always talk of it as past tense - 'It does not exist!' Only mention it when I am positive and talk in past tense.

I will make some more notes if I remember anything from the last 4 weeks, but I will report back after the Christmas break.

Never to Return

I really do think all realisations are simplistic, especially when they pop out at you. It's like one big eureka moment! BANG! And it's there! Simple!

I never did return to my *'Dear Diary'.* It didn't feel relevant at all after I'd decided in 2008 to stop focusing on EHS. This was such a big realisation with many aspects to it. My *'best decision day'* was about to appear right before my very eyes. *'A way had been found'.* Little did I realise how this understanding was going to pan out.

References:

[1] Mossop, D. (1990). *Phytobiophysics.* https://www.phytob.com

[2] Bach, E. (1930s). *Bach Flower Remedies.*
https://www.bachremedies.com

Michelle Townsend

Chapter 10

Best Decision Day

'When you stand at a crossroads in your NOW moment, STOP for a moment ...

be in touch with your intuition, your gut feeling ...

there lies your inner guidance, your inner wisdom ...

respond from beyond your mind ...

take the path you most connect with ... TRUST it!'

~ Michelle Townsend

'The moment you change your perception is the moment you rewrite the chemistry of your body.'[1]

~ Bruce Lipton

I had spent many years telling my story how it was. Believing the reality in front of me - what I was convinced it was - how I was responding to the electrical waves - what they were doing to me. I'll change that - what I 'thought' they were doing to me. The more I talked about it, the more I found it in my experience. Then talking about it more and more to prove I was right! It became my total experience, my reality, which I believed to be true.

I can't remember the day I decided to stop talking about it all - sometime during 2008. How desperate do you have to become to want to change your life? It was a sudden surge that flowed through me, a strong feeling, out of nowhere.

"I've had enough of this! I can't be doing with this any longer! I refuse to give this any more 'energy!' I can't cope anymore!" I literally stamped my foot down, addressed it and that was it! Enough! No more words to be spoken.

I already had a reasonable knowledge from reading 'The Secret'[2] and 'Ask and It Is Given'[3] amongst many other books regarding the 'law of attraction' - 'like attracts like' and 'we get what we focus on'. The knowledge I was gaining was giving me that little bit of hope that things would continue to improve. I was literally exhausted from it all, completely wiped out by thoughts rolling round in my head. I couldn't go on this way anymore. Hypnotherapy had helped tremendously, and I was continuing to train my conscious thought processes to help support me. No longer talking about it was very hard because everyone at the time kept asking ... *'How are you?'* So, I told my husband that I no longer wanted him to keep asking me how I was, or how I was feeling. I didn't even want to go there to that place of how I was doing; it was still raw.

I made phone calls to both sets of parents, close family members and people who knew about what was going on.

I said to them ... *"Please don't ask me how I am any more. If there is a problem and I'm not feeling right, I will tell you, I will let you know if there is something not quite right."*

They all agreed with me, saying ... *"Ok."*

I reassured them I would be honest and upfront and let them know if I was in trouble. I think for them it was a release and a sense of letting go. They had certainly got fed up with it all and I completely understood that. This also backed up my worries regarding EHS with both my boys not knowing what was really going on. I'd kept it from them, and I'd done a damn good job of it! They didn't need to own my beliefs and traumas; growing up being fearful or start believing electrical equipment, Wi-Fi etc, could damage them. Maybe it does. There is certainly information out there now that questions EMFs, but it's our beliefs about something that creates our responses. We add to the belief the more we focus on it, just like the 'placebo' or 'nocebo' effect of whether something will hurt us or not.

I started to use my music to help create and reinforce changes. I suddenly realised I had the perfect examples happening right in front of me and had for many years. Learning more about the mind, I became aware of something called *'neuroplasticity'*. I was starting to read and research more and more about the mind. Being a music teacher, I'd seen neuroplasticity in action. It always made me smile how pupils developed and remembered the notes on music. *'Surely, I could apply this to any new situations I was experiencing? I had a better understanding of how my mind worked now. This could be a way of thinking about it regarding my decision and what I had learnt through hypnotherapy.'* Neuroplasticity is the brain's incredible ability to change itself. It is the brain's ability to create change and respond to new information within its neural networks and pathways. We all have this function working within our minds. It just does it! Neuroplasticity is also known as *'neural plasticity'*, or *'brain plasticity'*. From my observations during teaching, I'd become aware of how we use neuroplasticity every day of our lives. We are constantly experiencing growth within our brain, and our brain just turns up to do the job. I continued to observe this during my teaching.

When first learning piano or keyboard, I initially get the pupil to become aware of the shape of the keyboard, the layout of the ebony and ivory on the piano keys. At first, pupils don't know which note is which - they haven't got a clue! No idea about keys, sharps, flats, naturals and Middle C etc. After a few lessons, pupils become more aware of this information, processing from reading the simple dots on the page to transferring onto the keyboard. Just like learning anything new really. I started to think about this process more and more and how it applied to life. Initially, pupils press a key with their forefinger, not applying all five fingers. A little bit like asking your gran to type on a computer, using one finger, their forefinger, slowly, unless they are a proficient typist of course. When asked to play five notes from thumb through to little finger, controlling each note individually, it becomes quite a task. The brain isn't used to processing the information quickly and easily at first. The fourth finger and little finger get in a muddle and usually don't manoeuvre properly. After a few weeks' practice, a few more lessons, fingers start to work individually for themselves - pupils know which finger to place on which note and press it. It starts to become automatic; no longer having to think about it. I started to understand more about neuroplasticity whilst teaching. I could see the process taking place; it was amazing me! The more I thought about it from my new perspective, the more I realised I could apply it to changing my thoughts. Plus, it was keeping me focused away from my old thought habits and fears, watching the brain create the firing and wiring of learning something new. It was fascinating observing these brain connections, which was allowing pupils to create physical functions, improve finger dexterity, the process of mentally reading the music and transferring the information to the piano keys. Normally pupils would think nothing more of this and just get on with learning the instrument, but this was, this is, neuroplasticity in action! I also started to think about other things too, like typing on a computer keyboard, or the mini keyboards on a phone. *'Think how quickly someone can type a text message. Their finger, or fingers, depending on whether they use one hand or two just flies around the letters. How is our brain processing that information?'* The brain had to create new neural pathways to do just that, and I could see that it did this easily with practice. Just like pupils creating a good routine of practice which is needed when learning the piano or something new.

Once I'd stopped talking about EHS, I would address any thoughts that popped into my mind. I started to notice the thoughts were becoming less and less. I would talk to my thoughts that were to do with any pain I was experiencing as though it was a person, another part of me. I used the pain as a sign of healing - reassured the pain and told it the sensations were a sign of my cells and body catching up with the new me. *'It's just my body letting me know everything is working out. I'm just working it out, everything is fine. All this pain and uncomfortableness is old thoughts and old beliefs releasing.'* The new cells were starting to fire and wire the new on-board system, the new belief, shifting the thinking. *'My body had lived with electricity most of my life, so why couldn't it do it now? I've never responded this way before!'* All these conversations would go round in my head, and I'd *'replace, replace, replace'*. I kept thinking … *'I have nothing to lose and everything to gain by thinking this way! If my body can create responses towards electrical items and Wi-Fi like this, it can create new responses! It's done an amazing job at building on this belief about electricity, so it can do an amazing job at creating what I want and live in harmony with it.'* I just kept talking myself out of the situation, continuously, repeatedly, over and over. I never gave up once; I had got into this new understanding, into this frame of thinking. I was determined to reprogramme myself, my mind and body. The mind/body connection exists, and I was finding out how powerful it really was. I was determined to let go of the old wiring system; get the electrician in; rewire the self. I knew my brain was changing. It was reorganising my functions, thoughts and responses for me, differing from how I previously functioned in the old habit - the old way of life before.

'All that we are is the result of what we have thought.
The mind is everything.
What we think, we become.'[4]

~ Buddha

I started to find the more I practised my new thought processes, the more easily my focus adjusted. It became easier and easier. Whenever conversations about illness arose, I noticed my views had changed because of my new experiences. Life was changing, it felt uncomfortable to talk about EHS. Little did I realise that these new choices and decisions would allow me to process the news I was about to hear a couple of years later. This was just practice, preparing me. It was a true blessing in disguise. One decision that would, in fact, change my life, moving forward, into a world of new directions, new thought processes and new responses.

A Way Will Be Found

The decision I made to stop talking about EHS was, in fact the best decision ever! As I was moving through this healing journey, new insights were being highlighted with regard to certain aspects of my mind and how it worked. We can create thoughts about anything good and bad. Thinking thoughts long enough creates beliefs. They become hard wired, habitual and become our reality.

I realised neuroplasticity allowed us to make new connections, learning new information, adding to our knowledge. It also worked the other way round. What we no longer require disconnects. No longer firing and wiring together. Here lies the 'If you don't use it, you lose it!' again. I suppose another way we could look at this is the age-old wisdom - growth is of course inevitable for all of us, we gain that wisdom as we go, developing and changing each step of the way. Focus on what you want; the rest will fade away.

Responding differently when in situations around EHS became interesting. How I was responding made a difference. The negative response or attack vanished once I started treating EHS as though it were a person - making friends with it, practising forgiveness, sending it love and reassuring it. That's when things changed. That's when I started to heal more powerfully. No response is sometimes the best, it kills the situation dead, highlighting that it is not acceptable, honouring the space and 'energy' to clear. Practising no response creates change, as there's nothing that can be thrown back, giving nothing but kindness or balanced 'energy' in return. Yes, accept it is there. Don't judge - let it pass - 'acceptance' is the key to letting go. Whatever negative situation is at hand, see 'IT' as a bubble of 'energy'. How we address 'IT' is key. Initially, I found it hard to not respond, but once achieved - seeing the power - I found it could be achieved again and again. No response is so much more powerful. I always remember from many years ago, where I didn't respond in a way the other person expected. I responded with kindness and forgiveness. I could have said quite a few things in return, got angry, but chose not to. The feeling it gave me, from practising forgiveness in that moment, freed me from the situation. I could really feel the 'energy' flowing through my body as it happened and as I walked away. It was unbelievable; it was so empowering. Almost indescribable. It would also have sent energetic messages to the other person to look at how they responded and change their 'energy', helping them to create positive change too.

'It is never what a person says or does that affects you;
it is your reaction to what is said or done that matters.'
~ Michelle Townsend

I was learning a lot from my journey through EHS - quite proud if I'm honest. Although totally debilitating, EHS taught me how *'energy'* can be manipulated. In fact, we all manipulate *'energy'* every second of the day by how we respond. EHS taught me how to respond around people and different scenarios in life. It really was a hard - but very helpful experience.

Everyone has different views on *'energy'*. Some people don't even connect with the word in the way I am describing it, but basically, it's physics. Physics is the study of matter, *'energy'* and the interaction between them. *'Energy'* is the life force that flows through all things. Everything is **'energy'**, both positive and negative. Every thought, every belief, every emotion, every body, everything is a form of *'energy'*, vibrating at either a high or low frequency. Frequency is the rate at which *'energy'* vibrates. Anything that is solid vibrates. It must, to maintain its solidness, although nothing is really solid. Atoms are 99.9999999% empty space (Rutherford, 1911)[5]. There is so much that we don't see around us, non-physical things that vibrate at a frequency. Remember - mobile phones connect via our phone number through frequency. I remember an experiment I did at school in my physics class. Apparatus was set up with five pieces of string each with a ball attached. There were two long pieces of string, two short pieces of string and one odd length. The odd length ball did nothing apart from swinging on its own. The long length ball was triggered to swing and after a few seconds, the other long length ball started to swing on its own without even being touched. The same applied to the short length ball. Both matching length ones started vibrating at the same frequency without even being touched. This showed that frequencies match and vibrate together. With the understanding I was gaining, I thought ... *'What if I see myself as 99.9999999% of empty space? That I am 'energy' in motion vibrating at a frequency? Surely, I can change that frequency to respond differently around EMFs? I can create the change through the power of my thoughts, perceptions, beliefs and responses.'* It's all about 'communication' - 'like attracts like'. My intention was to connect with the vibration I wanted to experience. This 'communication' thing started to make sense. When experiencing a negative *'energy'* response - no matter where it was coming from - I just kept responding with kindness - made friends with it - watched what happened

- became fully aware - became observant in the moment. It was almost taking a step back from the situation, as though external from it, looking at it from a bird's eye view. This created space to process the information, the *'energy'* that was being presented.

'Your energy of responding can be changed by YOU at any moment for the better. Your 'energy' resides within your responses. It's that choice of response to that person, that thing, that situation' ...

~ Michelle Townsend

Practise ... Practise ... Practise

As with most things, it's just practice. I was patient. I'm a very patient person, thankfully. I gave my body time to process this new understanding. I just practised new responses. My body started changing, responding and catching up with my new thought processes. Changing the thought consequently changed the response and reality followed suit. It's the same with anything in life, relationships, awkward situations and illness. If I had continued to respond and continued with the same negativity, with fight, EHS would have got nastier and stronger. Seeing 'IT' external to me became my choice - practising self-respect, maintaining and protecting my own *'energy'*.

Whether responses are with people, things or situations - whatever 'IT' may be - it's all the same type of *'energy'* playing out in front of us. How we choose to deal with it is our responsibility, our choice. This also brings back the perception aspect. We all perceive from our own experiences, our conditioning (as mentioned in earlier chapters), which in some cases isn't necessarily good *'energy'*. If we can train our brain to understand about *'energy'*, then we can start to foster responses that are for the better, not only for us, but for the other person or situation. This recalls the 'cause and effect' response. We may find there are multiple causes with multiple effects, looking as to why things happen. It is a natural human instinct, to understand why; but do we really need to venture there? Do we really need to know why?

Make things fun! We are more likely to experience positive results. I knew if I made these new responses fun, I would more likely respond by being blasé towards EHS and if possible, enjoy the process. It became a game, playing about with it.

During this time, someone highlighted to me to 'never own an illness, a dis-ease'. Don't own a thought, allowing it to manifest into beliefs, habits, or life. Owning an illness brings that *'energy'* closer, making it a part of you. You are much more than that. Yes, do what's required physically to help, but, first and foremost, see illness as *'energy'*, manifesting from your emotions. If those emotions aren't dealt with, we become stuck, blocking our body's *'energy'* systems, our meridians and chakras. Use the emotions as a signal to push and bring forward a change of new thoughts, new perceptions and guidance to help. Don't feed what you don't like! It's the old saying … *'Are you watering weeds or are you watering flowers?'*[6] (anon). Feed what you want in life. Let all the other stuff go. EVERYTHING IS ENERGY after all!

Just Become Aware

It's good to STOP for a moment and think about what's going through your mind, your thoughts and responses, no matter what the task at hand. Get back to *'replace, replace, replace'*. Consciously be aware, otherwise what could you be allowing to sink down into your subconscious mind each day? Down that rabbit hole? What is firing and wiring in your brain? We are all doing this day in, day out - all guilty of programming ourselves. At this time, I became aware of a fantastic docudrama called 'What the Bleep Do We Know!?: Down the Rabbit Hole'[7]. A documentary blended in with a storyline to help understand quantum physics. The film explores the nature of reality and the effects the mind has on it. An interesting educational watch.

Ask yourself - am I happy with what I'm making connections with? That sounds bizarre, considering electrical connections are needed to make electrical items work! Pardon the pun! Quite relevant considering my experiences, but that's how I got the deeper understanding. Ask yourself ...

- Do those thoughts feel good?
- Am I creating something I want or don't want?
- What new habit am I creating right now without even realising it?

Our subconscious loves habit - it's good at it! So, keep on keeping on and *'replace, replace, replace!'* We learn things naturally from our experiences but think about what we could deliberately direct. Let go of the old and bring in the new. It's how our mind processes new information - it's *'neuroplasticity'* - it can change and run a new program, so direct it! Just like I did! When I became aware of my thoughts wondering off track, I pulled them back and redirected them. Rather than just going through each day on autopilot, make a conscious decision to check in with yourself. We **can** change our thoughts. We **can** run new programs, just like updating an 'app' on a phone or device. Make creating and learning enjoyable, updating each thought. Enjoy updating your own personal 'app'! Because that's what you are, a walking 'app'! Remember to *'Practise! Practise! Practise!'* It will slowly become automatic.

"Like attracts like. Just be who you are, calm and clear and bright. Automatically, as we shine who we are, asking ourselves every minute is this what I really want to do, doing it only when we answer yes, automatically that turns away those who have nothing to learn from who we are, and attracts those who do, and from whom we have to learn, as well."[8]

~ Richard Bach

I was updating my 'app'. I'd found a way, but how was I going to maintain this way, this new decision I'd made? Was it achievable? Was it believable? Was it going to work? I'd seen improvements and my body was changing. I knew *'a way would be found'*. I just had to find it in me to maintain this *'challenging change'*.

References:

[1] Lipton, B. (2005). *The Biology of Belief: Unleashing the Power of Consciousness, Matter and Miracles.* Hay House.

[2] Byrne, R. (2000). *The Secret.* Simon & Schuster Ltd.

[3] Hicks, E. and Hicks, J. (2004). *Ask and It Is Given: Learning to Manifest Your Desires.* Catrlsbad: Hay House.

[4] Buddha, G. (n.d.) *What we think, we become.* [Online] Available at: https://www.goodreads.com/ quotes/ 1296640-all-that-we-are-is-the-result-of-what-we

[5] Rutherford, E. (1911). *'The Scattering of α and β Particles by Matter and the Structure of the Atom',* Philosophical Magazine, Series 6, Volume 21, pp. 669-688.

[6] *Watering weeds.* Quote. (n.d.). (anon).

[7] *What the Bleep Do We Know!?* (2004). Directed by William Arntz, Betsy Chasse, and Mark Vicente [Film]. United States: Roadside Attractions; Samuel Goldwyn Films.

[8] Bach, R. (1977). *Illusions: The Adventures of a Reluctant Messiah.* Dell Publishing Co., Inc.

Michelle Townsend

Chapter 11

Challenging Change

'Relax and breathe, relax and breathe, the space to flow, connect with ease.'

~ Michelle Townsend

'When you believe something, chemicals are often produced in your brain that give you what you believe should happen.'[1]

~ Dr David Hamilton

Just like I had somehow created EHS in my body, I had to somehow trust that I could create and bring back harmony and balance in my life. I had to believe that I could bring back the cells in my body that had already experienced life without the responses to electricals and EMFs. I had to reprogram my cells and their responses. Just like a stress response, which can be changed through our perception of a situation, surely the responses I was experiencing could be changed?

How was I going to work through this pain? How was I going to eliminate THIS PAIN from my body? After my successful hypnotherapy sessions, things were changing for the better. In fact, they were phenomenally better. However, I was still experiencing pain. It wasn't as strong, but nevertheless, it was still there. I'd made the decision to stop talking about 'this pain' on my *'best decision day'* but how was I going to maintain this moving forward? How would I maintain the strength to keep moving in the right direction?

I continued to create a deeper understanding of the mind each day. I WAS moving forward. But thoughts kept creeping in of - *'What if EHS comes back with a vengeance? All these positive changes I'm experiencing - will they remain with me? Will they stay and progress into a complete healing of my body?'* Questions, questions, questions! A type of doubt going round in my head. I had to find a way to keep my strength and focus. What was interesting and very different was there was no panic anymore. Times had been very challenging and still were. I really didn't want to go back down the old route of talking to myself like ... *'I'm in pain today. The mobile phone upset me yesterday. Then I went somewhere with Wi-Fi! Ooh my arms do hurt today. When is this going to get better? Am I ever going to get better? Why me? Everybody should stop using mobile phones. All the cell towers should be pulled down, and oh, I couldn't even watch TV last night because it was giving me pains,'* etc, etc, etc ... focusing very negatively and feeding it. Change was taking place on a permanent deep level within me.

I'd always responded with fight! *'Got to get rid of this thing, these sensations,'* but that was activating the very thing I was trying to avoid. My popular saying was ... *'Well, I may as well be a mobile phone mast in the middle of a field holding my arm up conducting the frequencies!!'* What on earth was I doing?? What was I attracting by saying this as a joke? My subconscious was taking this as truth. Especially saying this as a joke because it was said in a blasé way. I said it, then I let it go. Out it goes into the universal *'energy'* field. I was giving off that frequency, so what would I attract back? More EHS!

For a long time, I was creating more electrical sensitivity. Adding to it. However, it took a while to realise that one. We learn a lot from our mistakes. When asked if I was ok, I continued responding with ... *'Yes, I'm doing really well today, the sun is out and aren't the trees beautiful? Thank you for asking,'* ... or similar things like that. Not even bringing symptoms or EHS into the subject. My focus was redirected. I stuck to my decision. Even though I felt absolutely awful, down, depressed and shit! The only way I was going to change my frequency was to talk about other interests that were not specific to the dis-ease - moving away from the frequency of the subject. I'd now realised fully what I had been doing when I kept repeating the *'standing in the middle of a field'* comment!

These *'challenging changes'* adapted themselves over time, changing rather quickly. This place of adversity was proving to be the blessing of powerful change. I just had to keep going. Connecting with the understanding that things do change when you change the focus and your responses. The mind - body connection responds. *'How was I going to do this?'* I asked myself. *'Keep visualizing myself no longer experiencing any reaction.'* But I questioned it. I knew deep down this wasn't what was happening to me; it wasn't fully believable yet. Even though I'd made vast improvements, I was fully aware of this doubt and acknowledged it. This was about putting thoughts in place that would allow a complete shift in awareness. *'Subby doesn't understand the difference between reality or whether I'm imagining/thinking it, so I'll think it!'* 'Subby' was the nick name I gave my subconscious mind. It was easier to acknowledge and more fun! However, it wasn't just about thinking the thoughts, it was about feeling them too - getting to the feeling place as though it had already happened.

I continued seeing myself before I reacted to the electrical equipment, remembering I hadn't always reacted. I started by thinking about all the times I was well and getting on with life, enjoying watching TV and using my computer. *'What makes it any different to now? All that had changed were my thoughts around it.'* This however, created a lot of despair within me.

Real frustration. I found it hard to visualize something I had already experienced because I was grieving for that place free from symptoms. I was so desperate to feel normal again. I found it so hard going because I couldn't get to that feeling place in that moment; it was upsetting me so much. I was missing that old place, the Michelle free from EHS. So, this is where I started to play around with this even more - this mind of mine. Forget the stubbornness of it all ... *'Let's see how good you are at seeing things in the mind's eye.'* I said to myself. Because I'd had such positive change already, and the symptoms had changed - improving day by day - I decided to use this to work with again. I had to cling onto every miniscule positive I had. I was grateful for the improvements. *'If I can create these changes I have experienced so far, then how much further can I take this? Let's just keep going. Keep it fun Michelle!'* I kept talking myself round like I'd done on my *'best decision day'*, fighting with those demons. Although fight was no longer the option now. I'd learnt to let go and accepted I could create change - focusing on the phenomenal changes I'd already experienced so far. At least that belief was in me now! It was the route to shifting my vibration ... my frequency.

I had taught for many years playing electronic keyboard and other electronic instruments. Being on stage with those electronic instruments, speakers, electrical wires etc many times, so why wasn't I able to do it now? I connected with my 'past' positive experiences to generate positive thoughts. *'See yourself how you used to be, Michelle, visualize it! Your subconscious will believe it to be true! The subconscious does not distinguish between past, present, or future, believing all to be true at the time of thinking it. That's why it creates responses within our body with regard to what we are focused on. If I was focused on the sensitivity, I would create sensitivity. If I was focused on the past enjoying being around electrical equipment, then that was also true to my mind. I'll keep on with that!'* ... I continued on and on.

As I was dealing with this *'challenging change'* Mike asked me to go on a local radio show with him to talk about the power of the mind and the power of hypnosis. I was a great example of how the mind works and how it creates physical changes within the body through the power of thought. We ventured off to where the radio show was broadcast. The gentleman presenting the show was lovely and understanding. We explained everything regarding what I had overcome, and what a big thing this was for me being in the studio with all the wires, computers and electrical equipment. Wires were everywhere in a very small room. As we sat ready to be interviewed, I felt fine - great, in fact! We mentioned to the presenter that this was amazing that I could do this. He probably thought *'how silly'* but supported me. The interview went brilliantly. After we came out, I felt euphoric!

"I did it Mike!" I shouted.

"I'm so proud of you," was his reply. *"Look at all the new beliefs you are creating around this now! You are doing amazing! It's getting easier and easier for you."*

That radio show interview developed a very deep belief in me that it was sorted. I just had to keep going, maintaining and facing each of these challenges. I could finally do it!

I continued to put myself in situations where I was deliberately exposed to EMFs. It was important to find different ways to work with this. The only way was to let the guidance come from each experience on the journey, just like with the radio show. That was my choice. I made a decision, a very powerful one in fact. I brought back the determination I'd had to drive my new car. Even though it was so hard, I just kept going. It was a very gradual process. I was driving more now, so the belief to move slowly and gently forward day by day had been created. One step at a time. I asked myself ... *'How could I ever overcome something if I'm not actually doing it, experiencing the reality of it?* The answer is you can't! *'You've just GOT TO DO IT Michelle!'* Gradually building myself up and creating confidence. I had to have complete faith and trust that my body was going to sort this out for me. I had to dive straight into EMFs full force. If the *'energy'* of EHS became irrelevant, could I let go in one foul swoop? If something is irrelevant, is that a part of letting it go? What is the benefit of irrelevance? We can change our thoughts in any moment. It all depends on what is relevant to us!

'Face your fear and use the equipment regardless; the only way to overcome something is to do it!' I kept repeating to myself. I was still teaching music at the time, so I had no choice in that respect. I had to work. It was my job. Even though my responses were getting much better, I had to find a way to tip this to the 51% that would nudge me over the edge in the right direction. Then we would be up and running! It was just about changing my thought processes, using my imagination, just like when I was a child - like any child, the land of make believe. If I practised long enough and kept on going, new beliefs would arise within me, manifesting into a new direction. It had to, because that's where my focus was. What good was thinking in that old way going to do to the cells in my body? How was it going to benefit me?

My thoughts started to change around everyday life. I started to look at how I could manipulate situations for the better. How I could think about things differently. How I could change my responses. I think at the time it was the electronic keyboard that was the main item that I used to create the change, along with my computer which was also in my music room. Rather than leaving it switched off whilst teaching, which I had been doing for quite some time, I started to switch it on and leave it on. I also started to sit closer to it, nudging me into living with these EMFs. I would continue talking to myself in my head whilst teaching. I would be totally focused on the lesson, but any time pain raised its ugly head, I would address it instantly. Rather than getting frustrated and worked up that it was returning, I kept using the pain as a sign of healing. I would repeat those conversations in my head. *'You have lived life with this keyboard before, free from pain. There's no reason you can't experience living like that again! Look at all those years you've played this keyboard with total enjoyment, total feeling of calm within my body.'* I would go on and on and on like this. Reassuring myself. *'It's just my body catching up, it's ok.'* Using pain to create change. My focus had changed suddenly and EHS was slowly becoming a past event, a past experience, an old thought. It literally was the fact of 'keep on keeping on'. I was about to have more proof.

During this *'challenging change'*, family health issues were also in main focus once again. Rheumatic Fever, which had made Mom ill as a child, had now developed into heart issues. After being rushed into hospital, we were told she needed new heart valves. Mom's were now failing and blood was not being pushed around her body correctly. My sister was due to get married in August, and doctors said Mom would be in a wheelchair if she didn't have open-heart surgery, deteriorating quickly. It was a nerve-racking time, so a decision was made and in June 2005, Mom was admitted for major open-heart surgery. Both the main valves in her heart had to be replaced with titanium valves. Thankfully, the operation was a success. The funny thing was we could now hear her ticking! Mom's heart could be heard doing its work of pumping the blood round her body. 9 months later, in March 2006, Dad was also admitted into hospital. Following his major heart attack at age 37 back in 1986, Dad now needed a triple heart bypass. So once again, we went through the worry and concerns of major open-heart surgery in a matter of months. I distinctly remember being with them before going into theatre, followed by being at their bedside once they had come through recovery. The number of wires, monitors and tubes they both had attached to them was frightening to see. Dad became consciously aware from his anaesthetic whilst I was with him, which upset me - but I held it together, not showing him I was upset. All the electrical equipment around them both could have thrown me into sheer panic, with fears arising about reacting with EHS - but it didn't. I was amazed! EHS wasn't my priority at this time. My focus was Mom and Dad. This was another turning point which reaffirmed ... *'You get what you focus on.'* Everything I had been practising was working for me, I was now having confirmation. Dad's operation was successful too. Mom and Dad both had a long road to recovery, but this wasn't the end of heart trauma for Dad. His ill-health was to strike again in the early hours of 30th December 2017, when Dad was blue lighted to hospital. He was suffering heart failure. He had been experiencing funny sensations in his chest, wondering what it was days before. Once again, after the shock - Dad being like a cat with 9 lives - survived the ordeal.

Another Paradox ... another Paradigm?

So, let's say the paradigm that you find yourself in has created the paradox that seems to be true for you. There are plenty of absurd contradictory statements we can make about many things, but is it true? If thoughts create things, then what is really paradoxical about that? Can anything be true?

'Whatever your mind can conceive and believe, it can achieve!'[2] Napoleon Hill's famous quote is a great reminder here. Is this famous quote referring to the subconscious that does not distinguish between reality or whether we are imagining/thinking it? Definitely food for thought! We are more than our thoughts.

Stronger Challenges ... May 2009. It was around this time that Jake, our Springer Spaniel, kept approaching me and nudging me in my chest area. He was a very loving dog, but had never done anything like this before. He kept pushing his nose towards my thymus area. Why was this? I'd had many trips to the hospital over the last few years. It's amazing what dogs sense and tune into. We were about to find out...

We were away on holiday in North Wales in our touring caravan. It was the Tuesday of Spring Bank Holiday week. I woke up feeling a funny sensation under my left armpit.

"Karl, my armpit feels swollen under my left arm. Can you have a look please? It feels really weird."

I'd had a cold for a few weeks that had been difficult to shift.

"Maybe your lymph nodes are up because you are fighting that cold," was his reply. *"It is quite swollen though. It will go down."*

I'd also got a funny sensation in my chest.

"You'll have to go to the doctors once we get back home if it's not eased off."

This was now another thing to deal with! A trip to the GP Surgery once I returned home led to the doctor saying it was nothing to worry about. I was concerned it could be a sign of breast cancer because of the lymph nodes under my armpit, but he didn't seem too worried, suggesting it would eventually right itself. But it wasn't to be. I had various visits to the surgery in the next few months, but nothing was sorted. So, it continued.

September 2009. I was with Karl and our two boys enjoying a wander round our local shopping centre. We were walking around an electrical store which sold TVs, electronic equipment etc. I could do this now that EHS had eased off and wasn't my focus anymore. I suddenly had the most horrendous pain in my stomach. It felt like something was growing inside me, it felt as though something was moving and expanding in my stomach. No, it wasn't wind! Nor was I pregnant! I could feel something moving for a brief second. It created such a surge of pain, I suddenly felt ill. I highlighted it to Karl without making it obvious to the children.

"Karl, I feel odd. My stomach is really hurting, I feel weird as though something is moving in me."

Karl looked concerned. His obvious response was ... *"You haven't got a bit of wind stuck have you?"*

I responded with ... *"This isn't wind, it feels really unusual."*

I was holding my stomach at this point and started to walk slower ... almost stopping. I thought I was going to faint.

"Does it feel like a tummy bug?" Karl asked.

"No, I've never felt anything like this before." I replied.

Then suddenly it started to ease off. It eventually lapsed. Feeling concerned with what had just happened, I managed to shrug it off and we continued with our walk around the shopping centre. I was so fed up with feeling unwell. It had been going on too long. I just wanted to feel better, have more energy, stop experiencing pain all over my body. Something had got to change. It certainly was being a *'challenging change'*.

A Way Will Be Found

Just like the situation I found myself in with our car back in October 2007, I continued using *'relax and breathe'* whenever I was in pain. It allowed me to acknowledge what was going on in that moment - accepting, addressing and changing my thoughts around it, creating a new focus. The pain and responses from EHS had lapsed immensely, but not completely. I was experiencing many symptoms in my body; I looked ill and had lost a lot of weight. I just felt like I was living an existence not a life.

Dr Wayne Dyer's suggestion ... *'Change the way you look at things and the things you look at change.'*[3] became very relevant. When your life changes, change the way you schedule your life. Until you make changes, nothing is going to change.

'Am I happy to continue down the path I'm going? I have a choice in any moment to make changes - that has already been proven to me. By giving myself a schedule every day, I can keep myself occupied, focusing on something else.'

I persisted and distracted myself from what I didn't want to create, directing new focus, focusing elsewhere. The continuous persistence and practice strengthened the new belief system and a new reality. My thoughts and experiences changed. I started to notice less thoughts around the current situations that had been a struggle. *'It's just my body catching up now. Old thought patterns are releasing.'* I created a belief that the cells in my body were catching up with the new thought processes. It created a feeling of letting go in that moment to keep my focus, which was then being drawn away from those negative situations, attracting more thoughts related to a new place. Creating a wonderful new belief.

Visualization was the key at this challenging stage; it created the connection to new reality. The more I connected in, the easier it got. Any frustration of not being able to get to the 'feeling place' of *freedom* vanished. I was able to see myself in a body that was free from the symptoms. It was important for me to continue with the practice. *'Practise ... practise ... practise! Keep going! Nothing to lose and everything to gain.'* In the desperation of anything in life, I think we all feel like giving up, but in a good way. That giving up allows us to foster the 'nothing to lose and everything to gain' approach. I had absolutely nothing to lose by giving it a go! There was enough information out there that it worked, and building on the *'trust, faith and belief'* was all I could continue to do.

Just like the 'placebo' effect can create healing from a sugar pill through a belief that the treatment is real, the 'nocebo' effect can create responses of negative expectations and outcomes, thinking it will cause harm. Even a belief about possible side effects can cause the side effects to take place. Sound familiar?

Placebo is Latin for 'I will please', sometimes labelled 'a make-believe medicine'; whereas nocebo comes from the Latin 'to harm', where we are more likely to experience an adverse effect if we expect it. I had certainly done plenty of 'nocebo' thinking for a very long time indeed! It was time to switch to the placebo effect from this moment forward, programming the new way of thinking. When placing myself in situations to overcome EHS, I started to use this placebo effect to heal. *All these EMFs I can feel right now are healing my body.* I used the frequencies like a sugar pill, just like addressing the pain and using the pain as healing signals. I added a feeling that the sensations were good for me, creating healthy responses and healthy thought processes. I was no longer fearful of it. I continued making friends with it. I was using the very thing that had been causing the problem to heal the problem. Little did I realise I was about to have a major new problem. Everything I had learned from my experience of EHS was about to be put into use. Deep down, I still knew something wasn't right. Something else was there. My body was telling me that it wasn't free just yet!

References:

[1] Hamilton, D.R. (2008). *How Your Mind Can Heal Your Body*. Hay House.

[2] Hill, N (1937). *Think and Grow Rich.* The Ralston Society.

[3] Dyer, W. (2004). *The Power of Intention.* Hay House.

Chapter 12

The BIG C!

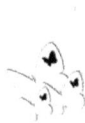

*'When we trust in ourselves to have faith in something
we can't yet see,*

*we create the belief that it is already sorted.
Connect with the calmness'* ...

~ Michelle Townsend

After experiencing all the effects of EHS, I'd sort of got used to experiencing pain. It had almost become a normal part of my life. Hypnotherapy had proved to be life changing for me, but something still wasn't right. I still wasn't well. There was the issue of the swelling under my left armpit. It was five months later and it still had not returned to normal. There was also the issue of my chest slightly protruding out on the left side just above my breast. I was experiencing funny sensations when I moved in certain ways in my chest cavity, persistent cough that would come and go, drenching night sweats, temperature fluctuating hot and cold and itchy skin that would drive me crazy - then sitting in the bath in the middle of the night and using wet towels to try to ease itching. I also had skin sores and lesions that would not heal on my lower legs. It was all getting very concerning. The thing was, I had already been to see the doctor numerous times, to be told I'd probably just pulled myself under my arm doing yoga and my exercises. As most of us do - we brush it off, we keep going, thinking it will go away and pass, but it didn't. It was getting worse! The EHS symptoms faded. Occasionally there were still the odd sensations, but I could deal with it now - I'd sorted my head and thoughts around it.

October 2009, we were away in London for half term.

Whilst walking in Westminster, I suddenly said to Karl ... *"Ooh, I can feel a lump in my neck."*

Karl felt it and agreed. *"You'll have to get up the doctors again to get it checked out. You're not right."*

I was struggling with feeling hot - then cold. I felt so tired too.

"Maybe I have a virus and my lymph nodes have swollen because of it?"

We were away in our touring caravan, staying just outside London. My sister was due to give birth at any time. I wasn't sleeping well because of what was going on. Then, suddenly, in the early hours, came the wonderful news that Karl and I were now an auntie and uncle.

"It's a boy!"

It was so exciting to hear this wonderful news. I'd become an auntie! However, at the same time I was stressed. I wasn't well. I was worried what was wrong. So many mixed emotions were flowing through me.

After we returned home, it was time to go and meet my new nephew. My sister was still in hospital. I was concerned that I had this temperature that kept coming and going. I questioned *'should I go?'* I'd had it for some time, but none of my family, or anyone for that matter, had caught anything off me for weeks, so I made the decision to go. He was gorgeous, such a little beauty. It cheered me up no end. My sister was aware I wasn't well, and it was lovely having plenty of cuddles once they were out of hospital.

That week, I ventured back to the doctors. I was given antibiotics, which I took, but again this didn't make any difference. Another return to the doctors and I was sent for blood tests. Whilst all this was going on, I was seemingly getting worse and worse. I now had pains in my stomach. I started to notice I couldn't digest my food properly. It was almost like the food was getting stuck and couldn't pass through. I had pain in my back, which increasingly became more and more excruciating. I was so tired. I had no energy. The bloods finally returned with the statement 'no further action required.'

Karl and I stood at reception in the surgery where I said ... *"I'm not willing to accept that! I'm not right! I want to see a different doctor now! We want a second opinion!"*

I managed to get an appointment there and then. The doctor checked me over and said ... *"No, I'm not happy, we need further tests with all of this. I'm sending you for more bloods and a chest x-ray."*

I went for the further tests.

It was shortly after, when I was sitting at home early one morning, I had an itch on my neck where the swelling had been. Obviously, my instant response was to scratch it. Suddenly, to my surprise, as I reached up to the left-hand side of my neck, in the clavicle area, I now found two hard lumps. I continued to investigate to then find three lumps! I instantly rang Karl at work.

"Can you come home?" I said ... *"I've found some more lumps in my neck on the left side and they are really hard lumps."*

Karl came straight back. It's at this point that I really thought I had breast cancer. The underarm swelling, chest area and now lymph nodes.

"If it is, we will deal with it." Karl said.

Had it spread into my lymph nodes? If it was a virus, why weren't the lumps going down? A return to the doctors for the x-ray results showed something in my chest cavity. Bloods were still not really showing anything, apart from the fact that my inflammatory markers were up. My bloods had been off balance for years, especially after the D-dimers scenario a few years before, when I had been going through EHS. So this wasn't something new.

By the time I attended my appointment for further tests at the breast clinic - the week before Christmas 2009 - the pain in my back and stomach area was so excruciating, it was worse than giving birth! I didn't know what to do with myself when it appeared. It would come in surges. When they hit, my goodness did I know about it!

At first, I was sent for a mammogram checking my left breast. I was then called through into the ultrasound area. I was scanned under my arm, around my neck areas by my clavicle and around my breast area.

"It seems like my chest is protruding out more on the left side. It's only slight, but I have kept looking in the mirror for months noticing a possible change." I said.

Lying there being scanned, I could see the faces of the staff.

I thought, *'Are they pulling faces because they have found something? Or is that just a normal response they give?'*

I asked ... *"Can you see anything? Is anything showing up?"*

"There does seem to be some clusters of swollen lymph nodes, obviously the ones you can feel in your neck area." Was the reaction I got.

The staff just kept scanning and looking concerned. Deep down I knew something wasn't right.

"We are going to send you through for a CT scan Michelle, and then the nurse will do a needle biopsy on your neck and under your arm."

I was just getting passed from one department to the next. Well, that's what it felt like. At least I was being given a good check over.

Next stop was the CT scan. I had to go in one of those tunnels. I got changed, drank this special liquid which would show up on the scan, then sat and waited for a while before going in. Once in, I was injected with the infusion and ... zip-zap through the machine. Once I came out, I walked past the room where the images on the computer screens were being looked at. There seemed to be a lot of concerned doctors.

'I hope that's not my scan pictures they are looking at!' I thought.

I continued past them to the changing rooms and got changed.

It was whilst I was getting changed that I overheard a doctor say in a very concerned voice ... *"We need to get this lady back in."*

'Mmm....is that me they are on about?' As I stepped out of the cubicle, the same doctor was walking past. He looked a little concerned, almost in shock at seeing me. That said it all.

'Was he concerned I had overheard him? Was I thinking too much about this?' I found Karl and told him what I had just overheard.

He said ... *"I heard it too."*

Karl and I were now getting really concerned. We walked back to the breast clinic area ready to have my needle biopsy.

The nurse who took the biopsies was lovely.

"Is this going to hurt, being as you are sticking a great big needle in my neck?" I said.

"You'll feel it, yes," she replied ... *"but it may not be as bad as you think. That area of your neck isn't as sensitive as you think."*

'Great!' In fact, it wasn't that bad at all, she was right, and she did it without numbing the areas too! I hardly felt anything as she stuck this big needle into my neck, then under my arm.

"Will they be able to tell much from these?" I asked.

"Sometimes we get results from doing these, other times we don't. It all depends on whether we can get a good sample." She replied.

That wasn't really what I wanted to hear, but just went with it.

"Hopefully, you'll get these results back just before Christmas. If not definitely in the new year." She told us.

"Ok, thank you." I replied.

We thanked the doctors for their time and then left the hospital.

Christmas came and went. My symptoms were still not improving; they were slowly getting more and more severe. I remember not being able to eat the lovely Christmas dinner Karl had cooked. I couldn't eat a full meal. I had to keep stopping as the food was getting stuck in my intestines; it felt blocked. Such a weird feeling.

January 2010 came, and I was greeted with a letter from the hospital. I opened it, thinking it was the results from the needle biopsy etc. To my shock it read ... *'Your operation, which is due.... etc etc. What operation? I didn't know I'd got to have an operation!'*

No-one had been in touch. It didn't even say what the operation was! I got on the phone straight away to Karl.

"I've got to have an operation! But I don't know what operation it is; it doesn't say!"

I started to feel quite panicky because the last time I had an anaesthetic, back in the 90s, for a Laparoscopy, I was unable to breathe when I came round. I had a terrible experience and fear of anaesthetic. I didn't want this operation!

"Ring the hospital straight away and see if you can find out what it is," was Karl's response.

Within a matter of days, I was admitted to hospital as a day case for a lymph node biopsy being taken from under my arm. The usual tests were done before having any operation - weight, height, blood pressure and bloods. I was so worried about going under anaesthetic that I kept asking the doctors questions when they came to see me.

"Can I have a local anaesthetic? Is it not possible to stay awake for this biopsy?" I asked. *"I'm worried I won't be able to breathe when I come round. Last time I couldn't breathe; I thought I was suffocating."*

They responded with … *"No, you need to have a general anaesthetic, Michelle. This operation needs you to be out."*

I was extremely nervous at this point. *"Will you please make sure that I can breathe when you bring me round then? I'm so worried."* I was pleading with them.

"Yes, we will make sure you are monitored; someone will be with you. Don't worry."

I had to accept this. What was lovely and reassuring was that one of my friends, Margaret, who worked at the hospital, was on the ward. Margaret kept coming to check on me and make sure I was ok. Karl stayed with me as long as he was allowed to, but then left, returning later to pick me up.

It was time to go down to theatre.

They got me in position ready and the anaesthetist said, *"I'm going to get you to count to 10 and you'll gently go under. You won't even realise; you'll be absolutely fine."*

At that, we started counting together … *"One…two…. three…fo…."* I didn't even make four I was out!

Next thing I knew, I started to come round; I was in the recovery room. *'I could BREATHE! Yay! I wasn't suffocating!'* That was the first thing on my mind. The staff stayed with me to make sure I was ok as they had promised me. I was so grateful. Back on the ward I was looked after well. My friend kept her eye on me, asking if I was ok, until Karl returned to take me home. I'm not sure how many lymph nodes were taken out that day, but knew that we would get some results very soon. Margaret pushed my wheelchair to the hospital entrance and waited with me whilst Karl fetched the car. We were homeward bound.

Days passed - a couple of weeks passed, to be honest - and we heard nothing! I was starting to think, *'well maybe no news is good news'.* Maybe the biopsy was fine and everything is ok. I was still ill, so we needed to find out soon what was going on. I decided to ring the hospital and get through to the appropriate department.

"Hello, I'm just enquiring about the results of a biopsy I had a couple of weeks ago. I haven't heard anything and am presuming everything was ok with the biopsy?" I was nervous.

"What's your name please, and I'll check for you."

"Michelle Townsend." I replied.

"Ok. Let me have a look and see what's going on with your results."

There was a pause whilst the receptionist went to find out.

"OH my goodness, Michelle! We need to get you back in as soon as possible. Your results had got mislaid and we need to see you. Can you get here tomorrow?"

'Tomorrow?' I thought. This seems urgent! *"Yes of course, what time would you like to see me?"*

An appointment was made for the following afternoon.

Tuesday 26ᵗʰ January 2010, we were sitting in the hospital waiting room. I was having a little bit of a moan, which is very unusual for me. I'm a very patient person.

"I hope it's not another doctor we have to see! That means I've got to repeat myself all over again, for the umpteenth time! Why can't they keep me with the same doctor?" I said to my husband.

I had seen many doctors over time, so was getting fed up with repeating myself. As I was called into the consultation room, I realised it was YET ANOTHER doctor.

"Here we go again!" I said under my breath.

He introduced himself and seemed very nice and pleasant.

Deep down my thoughts were ... *'Another doctor. I've got to repeat myself.'*

He told us that the other doctor was unable to see me that day, asked us to take a seat and went straight into my results. He had a lovely manner, and I did seem to connect with him much better than the previous doctor I'd seen, so I felt a bit of a relief, to be fair.

"I'm afraid it's not good news Michelle. You've got something called 'Hodgkin's Lymphoma' - a type of blood cancer, a cancer of the lymphatic system. Unfortunately, from the results of the scans, you have quite a few swollen lymph nodes in your body."

It wasn't just in my neck and under my arm, there were tumours around my stomach, kidneys and lower part of my body. The doctor went on to tell us that they thought the main tumour had originated in and around my thymus gland area. This meant that the scan I'd had just a few years before was probably the cancer. Oh my! Jake our dog must have known! The CT scan was showing large masses in those places. The doctor informed us that I would have to have a bone marrow biopsy in the coming days and a PET scan to see how far the cancer had established itself. This was needed to grade the cancer properly.

With this news, I instantly responded ... *"Right!"* As I slapped my hands on the tops of my thighs. *"At least I now know what's wrong, and I now know what I'm dealing with."*

As I looked across, my husband Karl just sunk down in the chair and broke down, as if like a balloon deflating.

I reassured him ... *"We know what we have to do now."*

I have to say at this point that it was totally weird. A peculiar feeling came over me, not one that I would have expected from someone who has just been given the diagnosis I'd had! It almost felt like a big, massive weight had been lifted off my shoulders, because I finally knew what was wrong and knew there would be a plan of healing ahead. I felt some relief. Plus, I had already experienced positive healing effects from using hypnotherapy. I also now had a good understanding of how my mind worked and I instantly thought ... *'If I can do it once, I can do it again!'*

I'd been ill for quite a few years with one thing and another - dealing with EHS symptoms - which I believe had masked the cancer. Doctors had been baffled really, especially when I mentioned EHS. Obviously, it had finally reared its ugly head. Had the EHS caused the cancer? I was still getting symptoms but nothing like before, so to me I believed I had healed that side of things.

We asked the doctor ... *"How long would this cancer have taken to be at this stage?"*

He responded with ... *"Possibly up to 5 years!"*

The look of horror on our faces! So, I had been walking round with cancer in my body for at least 5 years! *'Gosh! How could that be?'*

Whilst all this was going on, there was a lovely nurse who had been venturing in and out of the room. She came in to organise my bone biopsy and further scans. It all seemed to be moving so very quickly.

Karl then spoke up and said ... *"Can this bone marrow biopsy be done as soon as possible? Michelle has been left and messed around for weeks."*

My bone marrow biopsy was planned there and then for the very next day.

"We will get you back in tomorrow, then we will know more. We need to get this test done to see if the cancer has spread into your bone marrow, Michelle."

The doctor said it was definitely Stage 2 going into Stage 3, but checks were needed to establish the spread in more detail.

We returned home, where Karl's mom and dad were waiting with the boys. My mom and dad were on their way. When we broke the news to them, they were in total shock! They couldn't believe it, but I was reassuring them I was going to be ok.

Karl and I discussed what we were going to do about Aaron and Ethan. *"How are we going to tell them? How much are we going to tell them?"*

We finally decided to tell them both. At this time, Aaron and Ethan were 11 and 7 years old respectively. It was quite funny really, when we told them that mommy was going to have some special treatment and it was going to make her hair fall out! Ethan laughed, which I was so glad and relieved about. We made it fun, and we decided to do what we called '*mommy updates*'. Obviously, we only told them enough for them to understand at the age they were. Aaron was told more because he was old enough to understand.

I made the decision to also ring all my family and pupils that evening. I just wanted to get it done out of the way and I didn't want it dragging on over days, pondering how I was going to tell people. I just had to tell them as it was. There were many shocked people and friends to say the least. After all, I was only 39 years old and had just found out I'd got cancer. I told my pupils that I planned to continue teaching through treatment as best I could. I had to keep things as normal as I could, which turned out to be the best decision I made and a true blessing.

The evening of the diagnosis ... I distinctly remember sitting on our settee in the lounge just looking at my curtains. Of all things to look at, the bloody curtains!

'I've just been diagnosed with cancer and I'm looking at curtains! What the hell is this all about?'

Now this may seem peculiar indeed, but things began to seem surreal to me. I felt like I was in a dream. I suddenly had the realisation ... *'Am I really here? Do I really exist?'* I was observing the colours of the curtains, how they hung from the curtain pole, their texture and I started to notice I was just looking around at everything in the room ... *'Does this really exist?'* I mean, what a peculiar thought! But it was very real for me. It was almost like I'd moved into a time warp, where time stood still. Everything just seemed irrelevant, totally irrelevant. In this moment I felt complete peace. I felt at one with everything. I know that seems very unusual, considering I had been given this diagnosis only hours earlier that afternoon, but I was at peace. So, I just sat there really taking it all in and enjoying that peacefulness that was flowing through me. No tears, no negative emotion, no worry, no nothing. I almost felt that I wasn't there, just sitting floating so to speak. I was about to find out that these feelings were to continue in the days and weeks that followed. Connecting into nature and focusing on the detail of leaves, flowers, colours, textures, even the palm of my hand, just like I had done as a youngster. It brought back memories of looking at my hands as I transported myself to these places. *'Was I really here?'* What was important was ... this refocused me instantly to the simple things in life, letting go of thoughts that were causing distress. Simplistic but powerful.

I had said to my husband ... *"I don't want to go to bed this evening. Can we just sit down here and leave the TV on? If we fall asleep, we will be comfortable, so we will be ok."*

Now it wasn't because I couldn't face going to bed, or that I would get upset or anything, but it just felt the right thing to do. I felt comforted just sitting in the moment. I can honestly say that there were no fearful thoughts going round in my head at this point, I was just at peace, that's it! PEACE. Was this because finally we had an answer to what had been going on for months and years, or was it just a letting go, a giving up, an acceptance? I can only describe it as though something was wrapped around me comforting me. It was very peculiar, but lovely, and because of this I wanted to savour it. I felt safe. I continued to stare at the curtains and other things we had in the lounge - the physical things. It was almost as if they meant nothing to me. Obviously, they did, but in the big scheme of things, they didn't matter. Nothing mattered in that moment apart from the 'peace' that I was getting in touch with NOW.

Then, suddenly I found myself saying ... *'It's ok. If I have to go, I have to go. If it's my time to go, it's ok, but if I stay it's also ok too.'*

I felt a complete letting go of the fear of death. I felt in contact with me. That person who I'd been disconnected from for far too long had checked back in again.

A Way Will Be Found

FEAR!! That's it!! It's what I came to understand that evening. Fear holds onto the illness. It keeps us in the place we are frightened of. It has a hold on us. When we can overcome fear, our body releases the negative *'energy'*. It let's go! From that release, I understood there was more chance my body would respond to healing thoughts in that peaceful state. From that peaceful state, the cortisol levels would regulate, my body would not be on high alert and would have more chance of healing. This got easier for me. I was suddenly faced with death - how much worse could this get? I thought the EHS was enough to contend with. Now I'd got cancer thrown in my face! ACCEPTANCE!! That's also it!! I accepted death, and it's amazing what baggage I released. Everything became irrelevant. I was prioritising my life differently. Looking at life from a completely different perspective, through a new lens. I think it was at this point that I realised EHS was completely irrelevant now, reaffirming the *'benefit of irrelevance'* that I had become aware of in the months before.

GRATITUDE!! I brought *'gratitude'* in with this release, this understanding too. It was transporting me into the NOW! That's where my power lay. When in a state of gratitude, we give off the feeling of something that has already happened or having something; that's our NOW! It can't be anything else. That's what gratitude is! That's how the NOW comes into it. If I could release *'fear'* and bring in *'gratitude',* peaceful thoughts were more likely to penetrate deep within me and into my experience. I experienced all this that night, the evening of my diagnosis. The understanding of *'fear', 'acceptance'* and *'gratitude'*, I felt at one with everything around me. For those specific moments that evening, nothing was wrong. Nothing was off balance. I felt at complete peace, knowing everything was fine, whatever happened. I knew if I connected with the feeling deeply, I would be more likely to experience it in reality. Fear keeps us attached to the reality we are trying to release. Fear keeps us held in the negative *'energy'*. If I could let go of *'fear'*, I knew it would allow me to step forward.

It had been in the media that EMFs cause certain cancers. What I came to understand, as with most things in life, is that if we believe this to be true, then we will probably create that situation if we focus on it long enough. Now I'm not saying it does or it doesn't, but we most likely get what we focus on. I wouldn't be a normal human being if it hadn't crossed my mind as to whether the EHS had caused the Hodgkin's Lymphoma. I suppose I will never know. I don't need to know. What I do know is that the negative place I found myself, from the experiences of EHS, not communicating with myself, being depressed for such a long, long time because of my symptoms, could have caused the cancer. All these symptoms and responses were eating away at me. What does cancer do? Eats away at you! So not necessarily the actual EMFs themselves. I had been in a very negative place for a long time, it was bound to start manifesting in my body in some way or form at some point. If the EMFs had caused the cancer, everyone in the world would be dropping like flies from Hodgkin's Lymphoma, so my thoughts were never in that negative place, not even acknowledging it. Remember - we are electromagnetic beings through and through! Thoughts are electromagnetic and thoughts create responses.

It's funny how we think of different scenarios when placed in a desperate situation. It's ok to do that if it helps you let go in any way. I found I had thoughts about Princess Diana. She kept coming into my mind. *'If she could experience death at age 37, then I knew I was going to be ok too if it was my time to leave this time - space - reality.'* It was almost like ... if Diana can do it, so can I and it's ok. I found it very reassuring, extremely bizarre I know.

No matter what situation we find ourselves in, *'a way will be found'* to deal with it. Sometimes thinking of the worst scenario possible can allow you to feel free, just like thinking of Princess Diana's passing created reassurance for me. Death isn't something to fear. We all reach death from this physical form one day. My understanding from that night of diagnosis is we never die. How can we? We are *'energy'* in motion. When we are ready, we just step out of this cinema of learning ready to move into our next. The question is *'what are we learning from this life? What wisdom do we take with us?'*

'You are the vibrational writers of the script of your life, and everyone else in the Universe is playing the part that you have assigned to them.'[1]

~ Esther and Jerry Hicks. Abraham

References:

[1] Hicks, E. and Hicks, J. (2006). *The Law of Attraction: The Basics of the Teachings of Abraham*. Hay House.

Chapter 13

Trials and Treatments

'Don't let reality run away with you! Step back, take a breath. It's only your thoughts around that reality that throw you in a turmoil.'

~ Michelle Townsend

Wednesday 27th **January.** Bone biopsy day. I had to sign a consent form for the procedure as there were possible risks. I had to be sedated. Bone marrow biopsies are very painful procedures. Have you seen the size of the needle they use? A very thick needle is inserted into your bone. During the sedation, I would be aware of what was going on, but somehow not aware.

The sedation was administered, but I could still sense everything that was going on. I could hear the doctors talking as they carried out the procedure - sensing when the needle was inserted, as it was pushed really hard into my pelvis. I couldn't feel the pain, but I could feel being tugged hard at my lower back, rocking me back and forth. I was completely aware of it, but it almost felt like I was drunk and out of it. On another level of consciousness is the best way to describe it. I was brought back round from sedation and sat up. It was here where I saw the bone marrow that had been taken from my pelvis on microscope slides.

As I looked, the doctors said to me ... *"Yes, you can have a look. That's what we've taken out and that will now be tested."*

The doctors were quite happy for me to see and ask questions. I was interested to look. Karl had been given the chance to come into the room with me whilst I was having the procedure done, which he did - but as they started, he had to leave. He became overwhelmed, breaking his heart in the corridor. A nurse kindly took him for a cup of tea. It had all suddenly become real to him. Once the procedure was over, I was escorted back to a room where we were sat with the doctor. Apparently, I was quite funny, making both the doctor and Karl laugh with my responses. I felt like I was nodding off. Karl would nudge me to make me more aware of what was being talked about. The aftereffects of sedation were quite amusing!

Once back home that evening, I had complete rest. My lower back was feeling very delicate and bruised. Initially, it was very painful to move, but this eased off over the coming days. You could see the mark the needle had left for months. Almost looking like a chicken pox scar.

After the various tests I received over that 24-hour period, results were showing I definitely had Stage 3B, possibly going into Stage 4 cancer. Traces could be seen in the bone marrow - it was starting to show slight change. The doctor made a follow up appointment to discuss the results with us after I had received more tests. This appointment was to organise a treatment plan for me.

It was agreed that chemotherapy treatment would start mid-February. At first, they said Aaron's birthday, so, I asked could I please enjoy his birthday with him and start the following day. One day wasn't going to make any difference to me - we all agreed. I was informed I would need to have a 'PET scan' before receiving any chemotherapy. A PET scan is an image made of 'Positron Emission Tomography'. It involves injecting radioactive chemicals into the body to highlight metabolic changes that occur at a cellular level. PET scans pick up information that an MRI (Magnetic Resonance Imaging) can't. Not the best thought knowing you are being injected with radioactive stuff really - especially already having cancer in your body - but how else could tests be done to see the advancement of the dis-ease? The doctors needed to know.

PET scan day was interesting to say the least. It was like I was in a James Bond movie!

5th February 2010 will be imprinted on my mind forever. My father-in-law and I travelled over to Birmingham Queen Elizabeth Hospital for my PET scan appointment. Karl was unable to attend that day. I can't really remember travelling over there. Maybe my mind was so occupied with what I was about to experience, wondering what it was going to be like to have this type of scan?

I clearly remember walking into the reception area of the scan centre and being greeted by the receptionist, who asked me to confirm my name and appointment time. We were then told to take a seat and wait till I was called. It was very quiet in the waiting room. Only myself and my father-in-law were in there at one point. One other person came in - it was not really a busy place at all, which is nice to think, I suppose. After waiting for around 20 - 30 minutes, I was called in.

"We are ready to take you through now Michelle. Can you come this way please?"

The receptionist guided me to a room. My father-in-law waited in the waiting area. There were many side rooms in this small building. The one I was taken into was very white. There was a cupboard on the left-hand side and a bed across the back wall. Everything was just white! The doctor appeared and talked me through the procedure. He informed me that he would shortly be injecting a substance called a radiotracer into my veins. I would be required to lie down on the bed for around 45 minutes to an hour before I could have my scan, so that the substance could travel around my body.

"Have you brought some music to listen to?" ... he asked.

"Yes." I replied. *"I was advised by my consultant. He said it would take a while, and that I had to lie very still before having the scan. So yes, I have something to keep me occupied, I've come prepared."*

The doctor had a white coat to match the walls in the room, which made me chuckle! All I could see was white! The doctor prepared the cannula and inserted it into my right arm, ready for the injection. I always watch cannulas or needles being inserted. I need to know when they're going in. It makes me so queasy if I can't see it. Once the doctor had completed this, he left me.

"Just lie on the couch and make yourself comfortable for a while now Michelle. Try not to move too much. Enjoy a rest, listening to your music. I'll be back shortly with the injection. There's a button you can press there if you need us at any anytime," he said.

Everyone was pleasant.

I was aware that I was going to spend 2-3 hours in the PET scan centre. Only being allowed water to drink 4-6 hours before the scan meant I was likely to get hungry, but that didn't seem to cross my mind.

Eventually, the doctor returned in a special white suit, a mask and gloves on. He looked like something out of a Space Odyssey or James Bond movie! Almost like he was protecting himself from radioactive waves - well, in fact he was! The radiotracer injection was, in fact, radioactive! Radioactive! I was having a radioactive substance injected into me and I had already got cancer! It does make you wonder, doesn't it! But yes - radioactive. The substance, as I like to call it, was in - yes you guessed it - a white looking box that was locked! I was expecting it to hiss and let out white smoke as the doctor opened it - as you'd expect in a film. A special needle was all prepared, ready to inject into the cannula. The doctor got it ready and then slowly injected it into my body. He then placed the needle back into the box and locked it. I was then told to lie very still and try not to move for around an hour. The room was dimly lit. I was relaxing, listening to my music. Back then, it was like a small black iPod that you uploaded your music onto, except it wasn't an iPod, I can't remember what they were called. Nothing like we have nowadays, it was earlier technology. I was able to use it comfortably free from EHS symptoms.

"Remember you have your emergency button if you need us, Michelle."

The doctor then left and locked the door. This is something that must be done, as you can't go anywhere due of the radioactive stuff. I just had to lie there and chill. It was all very nerve racking, but I just went with the flow of it all. I had no choice.

An hour passed. I heard the door go.

"Let's get you in for your scan then Michelle. Are you ok?" ... the doctor asked.

"Yes, I'm fine thank you, just enjoying my music."

I was taken into the scan room where the large scanning machine was already humming away. It was one of those big tunnel ones.

"Let's just get you comfortable Michelle. We need you to lie on here and remain very still."

I was put into position on the scanner ready, having my body strapped into place. You can't really move much once in place.

"It will be noisy at times, and you'll hear different sounds coming from the machine. It's just doing its work of scanning, so just lie back and relax as best you can."

The scan lasted around 45 minutes to an hour. It's a long time to be perfectly still, especially when you have already spent an hour lying still ready to go in. You really have got to just listen to that music, focus on it.

Then I heard ... *"All done. We will get you back to your room to change and then you can get off home."*

After the scan, I was told not to go near any young children, babies, or pregnant women for 24/48 hours, as I was radioactive. The radioactivity had to naturally release from my body.

***

It was time for my first appointment, having had all my tests completed before starting chemotherapy. The appointment was to go through how the treatment would take place, what the treatment was about, the risks and my choices. During this appointment my height and weight were measured to ensure the correct dosage, so all could be prepared for treatment day. Karl attended with me. My mom and dad also attended the appointment, as we were told they could. I was offered the chance to go on a trial - the RATHL Trial. The treatment was to last 6 months (12 rounds of treatment). I would be on this trial for some years, helping to build up data about the treatment.

Even though the trial itself has now finished, data is still being gathered for people, who like me, were part of it. My treatment was ABVD, which is an abbreviation of the chemotherapy drugs Doxorubicin hydrochloride (**A**driamycin), **B**leomycin Sulfate, **V**inblastine Sulfate and **D**acarbazine. The success rate for this treatment is around 80%-90%. The RATHL Trial was testing how patients were affected by being taken off

Bleomycin after 3 treatments (6 rounds). A computer was to decide 'yes' or 'no' three months into treatment to establish whether the Bleomycin was to be taken out, continuing just the AVD for the rest of the term. Bleomycin itself can cause issues with your breathing and lungs. It can also cause symptoms many years after recovery. The trial was looking at how treatments could be improved. It was part of the trial protocol that I had to sign and agree to take part.

"In the trial, a PET scan given after 2 cycles of standard ABVD chemotherapy was used to decide what further treatment people needed. People with a good response (PET negative) were randomised either to continue ABVD or to receive AVD with bleomycin (B) being omitted. People who didn't respond well (PET positive) were given more intensive chemotherapy - BEACOPP.

Dropping Bleomycin for good responders after 2 cycles of ABVD reduced side effects. *Bleomycin has been used as part of the ABVD regimen for Hodgkin lymphoma for 30 years. However, it can cause long-term lung damage. The trial results suggest that dropping bleomycin and continuing with AVD in those who are responding well is safer but just as effective. Half were randomised to receive 4 more cycles of ABVD and the other half to receive 4 cycles of AVD. The vast majority of people (more than 19 in every 20 people) in both groups were still alive 3 years after completing treatment. 97.2% of those who had more ABVD and 97.6% of those who had AVD".*[1] (Lymphoma Action 2016).

Just before my appointment time, I was taken through to the room where everyone was receiving their treatment, to check my height and weight.

As we walked through, I was told … *"This is where you will be every two weeks for your treatment, Michelle. We will get you set up, then administer the ABVD. You can bring someone to sit with you, and certainly bring something to read, as it will be quite a few hours. You will be able to go to the toilet, but you will just have to take the monitor that's administering your drugs with you."*

The nurses were helpful and informative. All you could hear were the machines bleeping. The nurses were moving around checking everyone was ok. I just observed the room - it seemed quite pleasant. People were talking and laughing and passing the time of day. After the checks had been done, we then waited for my appointment.

All four of us went into the consultation room. My assigned doctor was very pleasant. I got on with him very well and felt comfortable talking to him. It was the same doctor who had told me I had cancer just a few weeks before. Around the ward, there were also the nurses I'd met over the last few weeks, so there were plenty of friendly faces around. The doctor explained the benefits, risks, and the protocol of the trial I was embarking on. Karl specifically asked about the risks and side-effects. He also asked about what foods I could eat. When you are receiving cancer treatment, you are advised to eat food in its freshest form. Sometimes you must avoid certain foods. Karl had been doing his own research and asked about the risks and possible secondary cancers which could occur and, of course, the prognosis.

Whist all this was going on, I distinctly remember everyone talking around me, but it wasn't like I was part of it. It was almost like I'd floated out of the situation, finding myself looking at a doorknob on a cupboard, thinking *'that's a doorknob! Am I really here? Is the doorknob really there?'* I became fixated on just staring at this doorknob. The only way I can describe it is I was questioning reality again; did I really exist? Does this situation really exist? Is this really happening? It was a peculiar feeling. Like I didn't belong to my body at that moment. I was totally aware of what was being said in the room, so I didn't miss a thing. Everything was clear, but I was external to it. No-one in the room knew that my awareness was drifting elsewhere - albeit a bloody doorknob!! It was almost a questioning of physical reality again, just like I had experienced on the night of my diagnosis with the curtains in my lounge. I seemed to keep having these weird moments, feelings and thoughts regarding physical reality. It's almost like something took over me to guide me - to let go of the worry, the fear, emotions and perceptions, and just flow through it. So I just went with it and let it be.

I was given lots of information to read regarding the treatment, but I never picked it up to read it until the day of my first treatment. Mike arrived that morning for my hypnotherapy session. We decided a session before each treatment would prepare my body well, as well as putting me in the right frame of mind. It is all about the mindset here. How we approach a situation. It was this first session before treatment where Mike got me to visualise the chemotherapy drugs as 'Pac-Man'[2] running through my veins eating all the cancer cells. My good cells would dive in the trenches out the way to keep safe. I also chose words as 'anchors' which created a signal to my body, allowing the drugs to flow through me with limited side effects. It worked great! This is where hypnotherapy was powerful! Perception is the key as to how we step through any situation. We have a choice in any moment. Maintaining a focus on living life, connecting with the enjoyment as we travel through adverse moments of our lives, can create a big difference not only to ourselves, but also to the people around us. It's the rollercoaster ride of healing. We must learn to trust. My hypnotherapy sessions achieved this for me - that trust. It's like I handed it over to the universe to sort out. I was able to let go of the reality just like that night of diagnosis.

On the morning of my first treatment, Mom and Dad came to see me. I was sitting in the dining room, taking time for me, before the trip to the hospital. Karl came in and handed me the trial paperwork.

"I really think you should have a read of what you are about to sign up for," he said.

I had a quick look but all I said was ... *"You know what to look out for, I'm not focusing on that, I'm not bringing it into my awareness. If I have any reactions I'll tell you, you'll know what to do."*

We made an agreement that Karl would be aware of what to look out for, as he had read all the literature, whereas I was focused on healing, well-being and not focused on nasty reactions or feeling ill.

I was very motivated at this time of my life, understanding that you get what you focus on, understanding how the mind worked. I had, after all, had plenty of hypnotherapy from experiencing EHS. That was going to be the blessing which I was so grateful for. EHS was the preparation; cancer was the practice. Making the decision to have a hypnotherapy session before every treatment worked wonders and kept me focused in the right place. So, I focused where I wanted to be and not where I didn't wish to be. Healing not illness. Not once did I worry about my boys - not once! I never allowed the thoughts to come to mind - in fact, they never did! I had already accepted that I was going to be ok, and that this was just my body catching up with the changes, just like I had done with EHS. All this in my body was just old thought processes that just needed a little help to be released.

Karl and I were ready to leave for the hospital. I said goodbye to both our parents. They wished me luck. The boys were already at school and arrangements made for them to be picked up at the end of the school day. I'd given the boys a massive hug that morning; they were aware it was my first treatment day and that mommy may be tired that evening. At this point, we didn't know what time I would be returning from the hospital. We had no idea how long this treatment would take. It was a blessing that my uncle lived near the hospital. Karl and I headed for his drive, so that we didn't have to pay for all-day parking - it was a great help. I can't remember the thoughts that were going through my head as we walked into the hospital, I think Karl was more nervous than me. I just saw it as a bit of an adventure which was going to make me well again. The cancer unit was on the second floor. We arrived at 'Georgina Unit' and went straight to the reception desk. Everything had been checked ready for the treatment that day, including a blood test the previous day to check my pre-chemotherapy blood levels.

The receptionists were lovely. They asked us to sit in the waiting area ready to be called into the ward. There were quite a few people sitting waiting, so we found a seat and joined them. We had to wait quite a while, but the time soon passed. Over the coming treatments, rather than sitting in the waiting area, we took a bleeper with us that notified us when they were ready for us. We would then venture down to the cafeteria on the ground floor. I was in a very positive state of mind throughout my treatment but found that not many people would talk to you in the waiting area. I found this very negative and didn't want to sit in there. This is by no means disrespectful to others in the waiting room, it's just how it made both Karl and I feel. The receptionists became aware of this over time. Each time I arrived for my treatment, as soon as I walked through the door they would start singing *'Michelle, my belle, these are words that go together well, my Michelle.'*[3] A famous song by The Beatles. The receptionists sang it because I was always very upbeat and made them laugh a lot. They said I was like a breath of fresh air when I arrived on the ward. I was, after all, practising positivity and keeping a great mindset.

A male nurse called us through to the treatment area and directed me to the corner of the room. The oncology nurses had gathered all the things which were needed to start my first treatment.

'Let's get this show on the road!' I thought.

A Way Will Be Found

It's only when in dire straits that we realise mindset is so important. The perception we create around a situation will most likely drive its outcome. It's where we place our focus. Keeping that balanced mind, enjoying laughter and living life to the full reassured me I could help my healing process. It was important for me to continue as normal, as best I could. Continuing with thoughts of *'I am already healed; my body is just catching up.'* Treating it the way I had done with EHS. Any dis-ease within my body was just old thoughts, old responses. I knew it could and would change, this would be determined through the choice of frequency I was emitting via my thoughts and mindset. I already had the belief that I could change the cells' response within my body. I had spent many years before doing just that. Those years had been a powerful preparation, a blessing in disguise, creating understanding that I didn't even realise I would be utilising in a way on which I was about to embark. The experience of EHS allowed me to tap into knowledge that I would otherwise never have connected with, making this cancer journey a completely different kettle of fish! I accepted that this was where I was right now and that's ok. *'It's just a space in time and it will pass, nothing is static.'* There was nothing to get angry about, no placing blame, because that wasn't going to get me anywhere. It was no good crawling up the corner of the room crying my eyes out, feeling sorry for myself - that wasn't an option - that wasn't going to change anything, just add to negativity and dig me deeper into illness, frustration and despair. Yes, it was hard having a cancer diagnosis, I just wanted normal life to continue. Carry on with my work, my life, and that was the way it was going to be! I wanted more, and I knew deep down within me that I could do it! Practising *'acceptance'* had freed me from the worry of what might and could have been, opening up many doors of possibilities. Those possibilities are there if we look for them - a big key to letting go. Giving in wasn't an option. Accepting and letting go allowed me to move forward with the right mindset.

I was becoming aware of more and more knowledge, holistic knowledge. Simple information about things like hugs. Hugs are good for you! Hugs, hugs and more hugs! I was certainly having plenty of them! Not that I didn't before diagnosis, but I was deliberately grabbing more of them now. It just seemed a natural thing to do in this situation. We especially found out how important hugs are during Covid times. Hugs release the hormone 'oxytocin', known as the 'cuddle hormone' or the 'feel-good hormone'. When in a place of vulnerability, sometimes all we require is a big hug! Hugs give us more than we could imagine, benefiting our mind, body and spirit. Oxytocin is known to help lower stress levels, lowering cortisol levels within the body, which in turn can help create a better chance of healing within the body. Those hugs I was receiving from my family were releasing feelings of trust and reassurance, promoting the powerful feel-good factor and healing within me. It was almost like I was holding on, hugging for dear life, when in fact it was what my body was telling me to do to help it. Hugs helped make me feel secure and gave a feeling of connection. I knew if I stayed connected, I would get through this.

References:

[1] Results of the RATHL trial were published in the New England Journal of Medicine on 23 June 2016. The full article is available at: **http://www.nejm.org/doi/pdf/10.1056/NEJMoa1510093** (Accessed July 2016).

[2] Tohru, I. (1980). *Pac-Man* [Introduced by] Namco Limited.

[3] McCartney, P., & Lennon, J. (1965). *Michelle* [Recorded by] The Beatles.

Michelle Townsend

Chapter 14

Journeys and Roller Coasters

*'Shit happens ... find the courage deep within you to
let go of things you can't change.
Let the past go.*

*Use it as an opportunity for your growth,
not as a place of regret.'*

~ Michelle Townsend

A s I reached the corner of the room, I was asked to settle myself in the seat. All the equipment was set up around me, ready to start. There were mainly female nurses on the treatment ward - only one male nurse. He sat in front of me and prepared the cannula. If you are unsure what a cannula is, it's a small plastic tube which is inserted into a vein via a needle. The needle is inserted, placing the cannula in place, then the needle part removed. It makes it more comfortable to move your arm when in place.

"I hope you are going to get that in first time!" I said jokingly to the male nurse. *"I always have to watch needles going in; I'm less queasy when I watch!"*

Probably not the best thing I could have said to him. He suddenly seemed to become nervous around me. I thought nothing of it as he proceeded. Then what happened was just my luck! First attempt failed … second attempt failed … third attempt failed. He had tried various areas on the back of my hands.

"Let's try just in your wrist area Michelle," he said.

"Ok, that's fine. Sorry if I have made you nervous by joking about it going in the first time." I said.

I then turned my right hand over, resting the back of my hand on the chair support. As the male nurse inserted the needle into a vein in my wrist, blood suddenly started expanding out under my skin. The vein had ruptured.

'Oh my! This isn't starting very well.' I thought to myself. By this time, I was starting to get anxious and frustrated.

"Can someone else have a go please - all this is making me tense?" I didn't want this gentleman near me any longer. I also don't think he wanted to try again. No disrespect to him at all, it's just the way it went. He walked away and got another nurse who then came along. She checked my hands and arms.

"Your veins are quite small, Michelle. Let's try a children's cannula size - see if that helps. The only thing with a children's cannula is your treatment will take a little longer because it is going in much slower."

Within minutes, she had sorted it.

"Can you insert the cannula for me every time I come?" I asked. She was lovely. Her name was Emma.

Emma took the time to talk me through the process of how the chemotherapy drugs were going to be administered. A certain order was required. Before the chemotherapy was administered, I had to receive an anti-sickness injection and a steroid injection. I just remember laughing regarding the steroid injection.

"You may find that you get a tingling in your bottom Michelle as I inject this in. It's quite unusual, so I'll administer it slowly initially. You may not experience anything, but most people do," Emma advised me.

So, the first lot of drugs started to go in. I was quite nervous, but ok. Sure enough, the tingly bottom thing happened, so Emma had to administer it very slowly to avoid a very peculiar uncomfortable feeling flowing to my bottom for all future treatments. Within seconds of the first dose, I could feel a tingling sensation around my body, especially where the tumours were - so I visualised the 'Pac-Man' doing their job and used the sensation as a sign of healing. Emma did indeed insert my cannulas every time I attended, apart from one!

After the anti-sickness and steroid, I remember a couple of the drugs being injected that were over quite quickly. They went in the order of *Doxorubicin, Bleomycin, Vinblastine,* then *Dacarbazine.* The first one, Doxorubicin, is nicknamed the 'red devil'. So called because it is the most toxic chemotherapy you can have. It poses many side effects, such as hair loss, nausea, and serious cardiotoxicity. It also must be administered slowly. If it is administered too quickly it makes you feel sick, getting a sudden urge to vomit. Even administered slowly, it's sickly. The red devil is bright red in colour (obviously), it also makes your wee pink after your treatment. I distinctly remember going to use the toilet as we left for home after my first treatment, and to my alarm I was weeing dark pink wee! Mike, my hypnotherapist made such a joke of it and started calling me 'Mrs Pink Wee' during my treatment. It made me laugh. The fourth drug Dacarbazine took the time. This was administered via a drip along with saline. The saline is used to stop the chemotherapy drugs burning veins. Believe me, when it started burning, you knew about it!

First Treatment Done! After a trip to the loo to release my pink wee, we ventured off home.

I said to Karl ... *"Shall we get some fish and chips from the chip shop on the way home? I'm starving!"*

"Yes, if you wish. Are you feeling ok?" He replied.

"Yes, I don't feel too bad to be honest. It's just been a very long day, with a lot to take in."

We stopped off for fish and chips. Not the healthiest I know, but it's what I fancied. We informed our local chip shop that my food needed to be cooked fresh, explaining my treatment - cooking it fresh from then on. I was very grateful. Gosh - those chips tasted wonderful! At this point I had no feeling of sickness. My ankles were very swollen. I felt like I was walking around with loads of water swishing around in my legs. I have always suffered with swollen ankles after having Glandular Fever at 17 - especially in hot weather. This was now taking it to the extreme! Karl's mom greeted us on our return home. She had been looking after our boys. They were so pleased to see me. There were plenty of big hugs that evening. We sat having a good rest, allowing ourselves to process the day and let everything sink in.

Saturday, I felt fine, in fact, I thought ... *'Well this doesn't seem so bad.'* I had a few aches and was tender where the cannula had been in place. I was drinking plenty of water to flush my system and the pink wee out! I just felt a little more tired than usual. Some friends came to visit that afternoon to give support. It was great! It took my mind off things and the last 24 hours.

Sunday arrived and I started to notice some effects appearing. I had been given anti-sickness tablets to use for the first few days following treatment, so I used them initially. Eventually, over time I didn't need them. I felt they were no use to me. I got up on that Sunday morning, but found I had to return to bed. I was experiencing severe pain in my face and jaw. I didn't know where to put myself. Apparently, this is an initial side effect of chemotherapy, which wears off the more you go through treatment - which it did. The initial first two treatments caused much discomfort in my face and jaw area. Karl kept coming up to our bedroom to check I was ok. I could tell Karl felt very lost at this point. I knew he was worrying what the outcome was going to be. What must have been going through his mind with those first few treatment days I dread to think. No-one knew what was going to happen to me. I had a good chance of survival and the odds of recovery from Hodgkin's Lymphoma were very high, but I also had to survive the treatment too. This is where we were now at.

Treatment days took a long time. The fact I was having to use a child's cannular made it so much longer than using a normal adult one. We would turn up to the 'Georgina Unit' mid-morning where I'd be taken through just before lunchtime, still sitting there at 6.30/7.00pm on the evening, finishing the last treatment. This took place every 2 weeks, and we had 6 months ahead of us. We planned it so that friends and family could alternate taking me and sitting with me. It also made them feel good that they were helping and supporting in some way. I would take crosswords, magazines, books and music into hospital with me. Most of the time I found I would just chat away and enjoy the conversations, the special moments of time we shared together, even though it wasn't in circumstances we anticipated. I watched the ongoings on the ward, also passing the time of day with other patients. We all supported each other. I found the support on the ward reassuring over the months of attending.

Each treatment required a blood test the day before to see if my immune system was able to cope with the drugs. Chemotherapy drugs lower, even diminish immunity to nothing over time. Neutropenia is a condition where the neutrophils are at a very low level in your blood. Having a low number of white blood cells weakens the immune system, making it harder to fight any infections. If neutropenic, it's possible that treatment can't go ahead. This is why regular bloods are required to keep track. There was only one time during my whole treatment that this was borderline, but following another blood test on treatment day, I was able to go ahead.

After my second treatment, I started to notice tingling sensations on my scalp. I was aware that this might just be the start of losing my hair. It was. I started to experience hair falling into my meals whilst I was eating, which is not the best thing - totally frustrating!

My hairdresser came between treatment two and three and I just said ... *"Shave it off! Be off with it! Just do it!"*

Both my hairdresser and Karl looked at me startled. *"Why don't you give it a bit more time, see how you go with it? You don't require it shaved just yet,"* she said.

Karl also agreed with her. Both knew how I had always looked after my hair and always made sure it looked in place. I was proud of my hair, but it was starting to frustrate me. I was finding hair everywhere.

"Ok, I'll keep going for a while, but I can guarantee I'll be calling you before the week's out to come back and shave it off!" I was right.

It was becoming unhealthy to eat. I really didn't want to eat my hair! My hairdresser returned only a few days later to do the deed and shave all my hair off. Karl and my hairdresser were really upset - upset for me - they were worse than me!

Once the hairdresser had finished, they both looked at me and said ... *"Oh my, you look beautiful without hair, you look amazing!"*

In fact, I did, I looked a proper G.I. Jane (1997)[1]. I quite liked my new look. I was so relieved to not have to worry about hair! There were of course the final very small stubbly bits to come out over the coming month, but it became no issue from that point. Phew!! Another step sorted!

Next, let's get my wig sorted! I'd been given all the information required. I had also been given the option of using the 'cold cap' during chemotherapy treatment. 'Cold caps' can be worn during treatment to help save hair follicles so that you don't lose your hair. They can be quite painful to use. You experience 'brain freeze!' I decided I couldn't be bothered messing around with all that, I'd got enough to contend with. So, I just let my hair do what it was going to do - fall out! Before treatment my hair had been in a bob style. I had recently had it cut shorter to ease me into losing my hair. The trip to the wig shop took place after my third treatment. I took photos to show the lady what I looked like before, so that she could suggest suitable wigs. Walking over to the shop, I noticed something different.

I asked Karl … *"Can I hold onto you while we walk please? I feel unsteady on my feet, I feel off balance."*

He replied … *"Are you ok? Yes of course if you feel safer."*

As the treatments progressed, my body responded differently. I had stopped driving my car for 11 days after each treatment because of this feeling of losing my balance when turning my head whilst driving. I could only drive 4 days in any 2 weeks. Karl had to start taking Ethan to school and we put things in place to help regarding the school run. I enjoyed my 4 days of driving. Each time I was out with Karl, I was holding onto him.

We entered the wig shop where we were made very welcome. I chose 5 different styles to try. A couple of them were longer hair styles, but these didn't seem to suit me. I decided on a bob style which was slightly auburn in colour. It looked like my hair before having it shaved off. I felt comfortable with my new wig; I did wear it quite a lot. Over the coming weeks and months, we had quite a few laughs regarding my wig. We had travelled up to North Wales one Friday evening for a weekend away at our caravan. En route we stopped to grab something to eat. It was only a small place, very quaint, and not too busy. It was nice to just sit and relax. The waitress sorted us a table and asked us what drinks we would like. I noticed she kept looking at my hair or my face.

I said to Karl … *"Is my wig out of place or something?"*

"No," was his reply. *"You look lovely."*

Whilst sorting our drinks, she continued to look. When she came back over to us, she commented on how lovely my hair was, saying had I been to the hairdressers that day?

I said *"Thank you. That's really very kind of you."*

It was in fact one of the nicest things she could have said because I was still very conscious of people looking at me thinking … *'She's wearing a wig!'*

I replied … *"Can I let you into a secret?"* At this, I lifted my wig up off my head. *"Believe it or not it's a wig!"* The woman suddenly looked shocked; you could see she was instantly embarrassed.

"Oh, my goodness, I'm so so sorry, I really thought it was your real hair." She couldn't apologise enough. We then went on to tell her my story - telling her of my party trick where I would whip my wig off saying *"Do you like my new hairdo?"* She laughed, but you could still tell she felt awkward about complimenting me. I reassured her it was the nicest thing she could have said. Karl and I made fun of most things to do with treatment. It lightened the situation and allowed us to ride the storm in a positive way.

My wig had to be cleaned in a certain way with special shampoo and conditioning solutions. I also had a spray which I applied that made it look shiny. It was great! Very warm on hot days though. On the days of cleaning, Karl had the job of going outside in our garden to flick the water out of it. Ethan used to find this hilarious, thinking the wig was going to fly over the fence into next door's garden. Thankfully it didn't, but we certainly had a few laughs about it!

On the opposite Friday to my treatment, we would venture off in our caravan. This was the weekend where I felt better in myself, but setting the caravan up on a pitch was becoming hard work as my energy levels were lower. As we reached the end of April, Karl and I decided to find a seasonal pitch where we could leave the caravan set up permanently. We would then be able to just turn up, switch everything on and just relax. We rang our favourite place in North Wales to see if they could accommodate us, but no luck. It took a few weeks searching, but eventually a seasonal pitch became available in North Wales where we originally wanted to be. We snapped it up quickly. As we arrived, we were directed to our spot where I realised we were right under the telegraph line. It was running right above our caravan. There was still the occasional fear I was having to address regarding EHS because I was still having the odd sensations. I started to become fearful and mentioned it to Karl.

"There's an electric line passing above the caravan, I hope I am going to be ok?" I said.

"It's a telegraph line; you'll be fine!" … was his reply.

"But what if it isn't ok?" I was doubting myself, not trusting what I had positively changed in me for a split second. I allowed *'fear'* to creep in again.

"What if I can't sleep, or sit in the caravan?"

"You will be fine," Karl replied … *"It's a lovely spot and we are on an angle with more garden area."*

By the end of April, our caravan was set up on the site. I worked with that telegraph line within my mind and apart from initial responses and feelings which my subconscious brought forward, it was never an issue. Once again, the adversity and facing the fear released it.

Just a couple of weeks later, after setting up on the caravan site, we became aware of another caravan for sale. It had a fixed bed and an end bathroom. It was a twin axle tourer. We currently had to keep making the double bed up in the front seating area of our current caravan, as I didn't really have space to lie down and rest if we had been out. Having a caravan with a fixed bed would allow me space to rest and the boys could still sit in the seating area. Before we knew it, we had put a deposit on this new caravan. Bank Holiday May Day weekend and our current caravan was fetched back from Wales, the new one picked up and a return to Wales was made. We never looked back from then on. I enjoyed many weekends recuperating there whilst on chemotherapy treatment. The caravan still sits on the seasonal pitch to this day! We have had 14 very happy years there.

It was around this time that I received the results from my second PET scan which was done 12th April. Results showed no sign of tumours. They had completely disappeared in a matter of 8 weeks! Treatment then continued with a more positive mindset.

***

On the day of my diagnosis, I had made phone calls to all pupils letting them know the news of my cancer diagnosis, but I had also told them I intended to continue teaching throughout my treatment. I stuck to my word, only ever cancelling one day's work in the 6 months, due to a bad cold knocking me off my feet. On treatment day, when returning home, I found I was becoming irritable. One of my pupils called Chris usually had his piano lesson at his home during the week but had been coming to my house since I had started treatment. I asked him if he would mind me teaching him on a Friday evening. I needed a focus to take my mind off feeling awful after being at hospital all day. He agreed.

"You will have to accept me as I am with my swollen legs and feeling a bit battered, but I need a focus when I get back home. Are you happy for me to teach you on a Friday night?"

Chris responded ... *"As long as you are ok. If you don't feel up to it, that's ok, I understand."*

Over the following weeks, I alternated teaching Chris at his house, then mine. On the evening when I was at Chris's house, Karl would drive me there and Chris would bring me back. It worked out great! It helped and supported me so much; I was extremely grateful to Chris and his family for putting up with me on those evenings. It did the trick! I was better focused on normality.

Further into my treatment, I started to notice various little things changing on my body. I suddenly became aware that my big toe on my right foot was becoming loose and weeping underneath. My nail was coming away from its bed. It was also happening to my middle toe. Thankfully, I didn't lose the nails. Eventually, over time, my nails improved and got better, taking years to improve but still not returning to how they were pre-chemotherapy. For years I had what looked like two big toenails on top of each other. It's only now, very recently returning to normal. Breathing problems were also starting to appear. Thankfully, the computer said 'yes' to removing 'Bleomycin' from the second half of my treatment. Any further lung damage was now removed.

After many treatments, my arms were becoming weaker. I noticed my strength wasn't there as much and I was dropping things more. It was subtle, but noticeable. Where the cannulas had been inserted into the back of my hands, the tissue was collapsing, and I was experiencing tingling and numbness called peripheral neuropathy. During one treatment, whilst Karl was sitting with me, the nurse kept coming over to check my saline solution, which stops the burning as the chemo enters the veins. As I'd had many treatments, I was getting used to it all.

"I'll let you know when my saline runs out, I'll keep an eye on it." I said to the nurse. Karl also agreed. Problem was, we got carried away doing the crossword and never realised the saline was running out!

Suddenly, I said ... *"Ooh, my arm is starting to feel painful and burning, Karl."*

We hadn't realised. It didn't register with us.

"Tell the nurse and ask her to check your cannula," was his reply.

Whilst trying to get the nurse's attention, I suddenly realised what the problem was. It was becoming excruciating.

"Oh my God! My saline has run right out! Quick! Get the nurse - it's burning me!"

Karl got up and fetched the nurse, who quickly resolved the problem.

"You didn't keep a close eye on that, did you?" She said. Chuckling at the same time.

"No, we didn't, did we. My fault completely," I replied.

That incident caused a bit of damage to the back of my left hand, which you can still see to this day. The tissue certainly collapsed between my tendons.

It was shortly after this episode that I was starting to get fed up with the treatment - it was taking its toll on me. On my return to the hospital two weeks later, I pleaded with the Nurse/Manager, Ros, who was the Haemato-Oncology Nurse Specialist. I asked for a PICC line to be fitted so that I didn't have to have any more treatments via a cannula in the back of my hands.

"No, you've come this far Michelle, you don't need one!" ... was her response.

"I don't want anymore; it's hurting my arms so much," I replied.

"No; we will find another area higher up your arm Michelle. It doesn't need to be on the back of your hand; we can move the cannula higher up for you. You only have another 3 treatments left. PICC lines are hard to look after. You are so near the end now; you can do this," She insisted.

I reluctantly agreed, feeling deflated. *"Ok, as long as it's not going in the back of my hands. I have no veins left; they are giving up in my hands!"*

This was the only time that I felt extremely low during chemotherapy. It was getting me down. It had been a journey and a half. Thankfully, Ros was right with her guidance, which I'm eternally thankful for - I made it through the next 3 treatments.

Throughout my cancer journey, I certainly learnt who my true friends were. The people who we thought would be there for us distanced themselves. One of the loneliest places was the school gates. There was a small number of people who offered their support, asking how things were, but many avoided talking to us. I understand that sometimes people don't know what to say in situations like this, but all you want, as someone going through cancer, is for people to treat you normally. The frustration of this peaked on the day before my last treatment.

"Fuck it! I've had enough of this. It's a hot summer's day and I am going down the school without my wig on! I'll show 'em! I don't care what they think! Will you come with me?" I suddenly said to Karl.

"Yes, of course I will," he replied.

School term finished that day. We parked up and both of us walked towards the school gates hand in hand. People were shocked to see me this way; you could see them staring and still none of them spoke or approached me apart from the small number of people who had supported us. I hated the school gates for this reason! I was partly glad that I was unable to drive during most of my treatment, as I didn't have to face the energy around this.

23rd July 2010 was my last treatment day. It was quite special. Up at the crack of dawn, ready to travel to Shugborough

Estate, in Staffordshire. Mike, Karl and I had a hot air balloon flight to catch. It was Mike's 40th Birthday present from us. Mike had surprised me with a Rally Driving Experience which was planned for a later date, but right now my last treatment day was a milestone, so we marked it with this uplifting experience - (pardon the pun!) The weather was perfect. It was so peaceful up there, floating over the landscape. So quiet. It truly was amazing. All arranged to fit in with my last visit to the hospital. I really do remember the day in such a positive way. It was now my chance to float into the next part of my healing journey.

A Way Will Be Found

No matter what adversity is thrown at us or what we have to sort out, we deal with it. Do we really need to worry about all these obstacles? Do we have to sort it out all in one go? No! We don't. Where does this come from, with regard to having to sort everything there and then? Can we not learn to trust the process? The steps we go through, the journey of adversity, the obstacles placed in our way. Can we not understand that time allows us to do that? The treatment journey was just that; a process. I had to learn to take each step at a time, otherwise I would end up stressing myself out for no reason at all. I didn't always know the answer right in the moment, I didn't always see or feel the guidance coming through. I just had to trust the process. If I'd have had all the answers, how would I have approached this journey? Would I have done things differently? No. I don't think I would have. What this experience taught me was to trust in me, trust it was going to work out, trust I would know what to do when adversity was thrown in my face. This strengthened me so much. It brought forward the *'trust, faith and belief'* that I needed. There was no other way. It was all I had.

References:

[1] *G.I. Jane* (1997). Moore, D. *Navy SEALs* (Film). Produced by Largo Entertainment, Scott Free Productions, and Caravan Pictures. Distributed by Hollywood Pictures.

Michelle Townsend

Chapter 15

Trust ... Faith ... Belief

'When you can't see the road clearly ahead ...
Have TRUST, FAITH and BELIEF you will be
guided at the next turn.'

~ Michelle Townsend

Trust ~ Trust you will be guided every step of the way.

Faith ~ Blind faith. Even though you can't see the outcome, have faith in the possibilities.

Belief ~ Create the belief deep within you; it is already sorted.

These three words proved to be extremely important to me back in 2010. They were what got me through my cancer journey. Created during a hypnotherapy session, I chose these three words as 'anchors' to work with. They felt right to me. This is another technique I used. I repeated them over and over. Just like the *'relax and breathe'* that had worked so powerfully for me when experiencing EHS. I had a strong belief in using words that reflected what was required in times of need. I applied them when in pain or when thoughts of worry, concern or fear crept in. I worked with them in moments of adversity and nipped feelings and responses in the bud straight away. *'Relax and breathe'* remained strong within my mind of how effective it was. I even use it to this day, applying whenever I feel the need to - using the technique in all aspects of my life. This approach worked extremely well; it created a strong belief. I trusted it. Had faith in it. I felt reassured and able to keep the perspective of healing flowing through every part of me.

'Trust ... faith ... belief' became as strong if not stronger - than the *'relax and breathe'* statement. I reiterated it so many times to reassure myself. I felt a calmness flow through me. The understanding that came from these words resonated through every cell.

During my cancer journey, Mike always kept me focused on wellness - that I was already healed - as though it was a forgone conclusion. Any time I would mention cancer in front of him he would very quickly change the subject matter, redirecting my focus and thoughts to wellness, enjoyment and being in the 'now' moment. He wouldn't allow me to talk about cancer in any way. This is far from not accepting what was going on. I had accepted it. It's about focusing on where I wanted to be - healthy, well and living life to the best I could. Understanding the 'law of attraction' continued to help here - 'we get what we focus on!'

After working through the pain, discomfort, thought processes and frustration, I was starting to make further progress in my mind - my mind felt stronger. My *'best decision day'* was by far a total eureka moment! I wasn't feeding that *'energy'* anymore. I wasn't feeding those responses. The *'energy'* that I was feeding was where I wanted to be and experience. I had connected into a new reality in effect. Having this realisation with the EHS was ground-breaking! That's the *'blind faith'* part. Not seeing the reality of it initially, but having complete faith. It was there to tap into - to extend into - if I chose to do so - choosing to use the pain to create the healing. That *'challenging change'* created the deep understanding that my cells and responses were indeed catching up with my thoughts,

I was living proof at this point that I was *'creating my own reality'*. I was reading the 'Seth Speaks'[1] book by Jane Roberts, which gave me understanding regarding the nature of reality and death, letting go of the fear of death. It was reassuring. After all, what was reality? My new perspective gave me that very deep understanding of the vastness within ourselves - it exists. Thus, creating yet another superb eureka moment.

I started to question things, lots of things. I had already got a strong belief within me that we can change and heal our body through the power of thought. Cancer diagnosis was traumatic, but not like I'd expect it to be. I know that sounds completely bizarre. I had experienced such an horrendous time with EHS - what could get any worse? I had made good progress diminishing the effects of EHS responses. They were very minimal now, so I knew I could apply this understanding again - helping me get through this next obstacle that had been placed in front of me. The new approach was already there waiting to be used. I had everything to gain and nothing to lose from thinking in this way. If it didn't work, then so be it. At least I had tried. Remembering I'd had great responses and change in my physical body from applying this approach before, I decided I **would** do it again! I **could** do it again! It was almost as though EHS had prepared me for the cancer journey. Yep - preparation! But this time it was different - completely different.

I was in no way going to allow thoughts to take over me, as I knew and understood that *'I am more than my thoughts.'* Yes, thoughts of ... *'did the EHS cause the cancer?'* ... crept into my mind many times, but I didn't allow those thoughts to take over me. I was fostering the approach that would empower me rather than self-sabotage me. I had secretly challenged my mind to help heal my body again! These experiences were pushing me to the extremes, so I created as much fun as I could around the techniques and words, which made it a more positive experience. I really do think that's why these three words became so powerful as I said them in my mind. What was this teaching me in life? About life? Whatever it was, it was certainly extremely powerful!

A Way Will Be Found

What was so special about *'trust, faith and belief?'* Why and how did I come to use these words in such a powerful way? Here's how I perceived them.

TRUST...

I had gone through life for a long time not trusting myself, not trusting my inner guidance, always wanting external validation. I can still be guilty of that now, but I think we are all guilty of this in some way or form. I lacked confidence in making decisions. It was almost like I had to get permission to do something. EHS had tipped me so far over the edge to find myself that I had to start taking the guidance from within. I had to start standing my ground with ME! Taking control of my mind was the big realisation. Understanding that I could create change and could direct my life where I wanted it to go. I had never had that deep understanding before. It was a massive shake up for me at the time. Learning to TRUST in myself was a belief I had to face head on. This TRUST came from using the words *'Relax and Breathe'* over and over. The responses I was receiving back from my body were mind blowing! These responses gave me the realisation that I COULD trust in me. I COULD direct my life where I wanted it to go. Creating that deep understanding. Just a little effort and persistence is all that was required. Understanding how our cheeky little monkey brain, 'the subconscious' works, helped.

FAITH...

Initially, this FAITH part took a while to adjust to. I asked questions in my mind ... *'How can I have faith in something that I can't yet see? How can I believe in something that isn't yet there?'* To put it bluntly, I couldn't. That's the whole *'blind faith'* thing. Persistence is faith! That's where I had to place my trust.

It was back to the ... *'Let's give it a go, I have nothing to lose and everything to gain'* scenario. Back to the *'relax and breathe'.* There was absolutely no way of proving that the situation I was wanting would come to fruition, but with the right thought processes, mindset, and understanding that thoughts create reality, I had absolutely everything to gain. FAITH got me focused on the qualities of life that allow enjoyment. This BLIND FAITH seemed to allow me to let go of the worrying situation and propelled me into the direction I was focusing on. It certainly allowed me to free up my thoughts, my mind, letting me live life during a major trauma. I started to experience situations around me that matched my thoughts. It's how focus works. We get what we focus on. If you become aware and tune in to what's going on around you, you start to notice things appearing in your life that match your thought process. Giving off the frequency of the desired action, situations must match up. This was also helpful in allowing that connection into the enjoyment aspect of life. Even if things didn't work out as planned, at least it was giving me that freedom from concern and worry - that breathing space. Savouring the NOW moments. Either way, it was a WIN WIN!

BELIEF...

Our beliefs come from our experiences and our practised thoughts. Thinking a particular thought over and over, repeating it and practising it, creates beliefs deep within our subconscious. We then find ourselves feeling, responding and talking from our place of belief - reaffirming what we believe to be true in reality, thus showing up in our life. This could include self-defeating behaviour or a wonderful appetite for living. It solely depends on your belief.

'No one is ready for a thing until he believes he can acquire it. The state of mind must be BELIEF, not mere hope or wish.'[2]

~ Napoleon Hill

Looking back at the *'trust and faith'* part, you can start to see how this could make change in your life. In fact, it most probably will. That's how it works - its physics, it's frequency! Furthermore, any belief is a perception of reality. We create our perception through our thoughts and experiences. Perception is reality. So, if perception is reality and perception is created through our focus, our thoughts and our experiences, then surely, we can change our reality?

There are always realities we don't like - realities we don't want to see - but with this deeper understanding, could we adjust it? Could we direct it just like a director directs a movie? This is a good metaphor to use. I imagined I was directing my own movie. I was the director, the producer, determining what's on the screen of my life. I created the belief of looking at life like a movie theatre. I started to understand that nothing would come into my life unless there was a reason for it, a learning, a teaching. You can *'fear'* your fears or future outcomes, or you can choose to use them to live effectively. I was now choosing the effectively option!

The movie theatre metaphor is helpful regarding the *'trust ... faith ... belief'* technique. Asking questions such as. *'How am I dealing with this situation? Can I change my approach? What's this showing me?'* That's how I got my head around it.

It was also important when working with the *'belief'* part to believe that the situation was already sorted. We have all experienced the feeling of calmness and relief when we say, *'it will sort'* or *'it's sorted'.* Acknowledging this opens doors and circumstances change. Your perception changes to a state, a frequency of finding a resolution, rather than focusing on the problem. It allows that particular thing or situation to fall into place. It's a type of letting go technique. As you let go, the *'trust and faith'* seem to lock into place from that decision. The *'belief'* then, more than likely becomes a foregone conclusion. You believe it's sorted, so you *'trust'* and have *'faith'* in it. Sounds complicated, but is purely simple.

Writing this book has highlighted to me what I went through back then. I'm quite proud of how I dealt with it all. I was very strong minded, thanks to hypnotherapy. As life goes on, the trauma softens. You forget a lot of it - flowing into the next routine. But it is these statements of *'relax and breathe'* and *'trust ... faith ... belief'* that remain with me.

The writing journey of recalling all the experiences, realising the trauma and the near brush with death, brings forward a connection to *'gratitude'*. This also brings forward the realisation of how quickly we can change and move into these new routines, and shows the complexity, yet the simplicity, of change. They say time heals, it certainly does.

Connecting my mind into a place of healing was amazing! No longer feeling lost, achieving *'a way to be found'*. Just having that ... *'trust, faith and belief'.*

References:

[1] Roberts, J. (1994). *Seth Speaks*. New World Library.

[2] Hill, N. (1973). *Think and Grow Rich*. Ralston Society.

Michelle Townsend

Chapter 16

It's OK

'Gratitude' ... STOP! - Take time to explore what's around you.

See, connect with the simplicity. Notice the colours,
the textures, the detail.

Gratitude in its simplest form ... creates a world
to be grateful for'.

~ Michelle Townsend

My mind work was getting good. I'd got good techniques such as *'relax and breathe', 'practise ... practise ... practise', 'trust ... faith ... belief'* and addressing it with *'it's ok'* - which was working very well ... but I needed more. *'It's ok'* started to develop into something stronger. Over the years, I'd always been concerned with ... *'Was I doing this technique correctly or that technique correctly?'* Always searching for guidance of the right way, searching for reassurance - childhood programming here, looking for reassurance for me. Noticing my own patterns and habits became the key to adapting and personalising what I needed. I'd say to myself ... *'That's a good idea, but let's do it this way approach. I'm living my life, so why should I need an approach to be a certain way? If it wasn't working fully, why not adapt it ... develop it? I'm more likely to stick with it and use it on a consistent basis then.'* So that's what I did!

Mike had started me on something similar to *'it's ok'* technique years before with EHS, so I developed it further, made it my own, adjusting it, manipulating it. I started working with my NOW moment. Shifting to a place that created a feeling of *'it's ok'.* In that NOW moment I was no longer in my past, nor was I in my future. Thoughts related to the past and future were allowing my mind to roam into negative territory. I needed to change them. *'If I can foster an attitude of being right here, right now and feel the gratitude for what I can see, hear and feel in any moment, I can allow the 'TRUST ... FAITH ... BELIEF' to shift me.'* Working through the feelings of having EHS and cancer had proved difficult. By putting in place a structured technique, adapted by myself, allowed healthy thoughts to flow through my mind. This made a new perspective instantly accessible, shifting me into that NOW moment in a positive way, easily. Refocusing was so important.

September 2010 brought the results of my chemotherapy treatment. Had it been successful? Did I require more treatment?

I had reached my 40th birthday back in May. I'd never had a big birthday party celebration - apart from my wedding day. So, it was planned that a special 40th birthday party would take place in September, after treatment had finished. My party was planned for Saturday 18th September, at a local golf club. The appointment for my results was the following Tuesday. Something to look forward to, even though it was a nerve-racking time.

Karl and I arranged a fancy-dress party. I just wanted to laugh and giggle and make things as much fun as possible, enjoying every NOW moment. It was fun deciding what to dress up as. With my beliefs being on a holistic level, I decided to dress up as a fairy with my jar of fairy dust. I still had no hair;

it was just starting to grow back, so my wig had to be part of my outfit. Karl dressed up as the Lone Ranger, Aaron as David Crockett and Ethan as Luke Skywalker. Everyone turned up in fantastic outfits. It was just fab! I loved it! Every time someone arrived, there were fits of laughter. Looking around the room, I could see Kevin and Perry, Gladiator, Jail Escapees, Top Gun Maverick, Mexicans, Egyptians, Army, Pink Ladies from Grease, Rapunzel, Teletubbies, Jack Sparrow etc. So many had made such a fantastic effort. Karl had created boards in the entrance and around the room for people to look at photos of my life. Such happy memories. Everyone thoroughly enjoying themselves.

A competition took place for the best outfit - best female, male and child. The bar staff chose the winner. My sister won with her fabulous Mary Poppins outfit. Chris, who had been so supportive on all those Friday nights after treatment, won, attending as a Dairylea Triangle. He later informed me that he had only made the outfit the night before! But in my eyes, all the children won - they looked fabulous! The celebrations also included Karl's mom and dad's 40th Wedding Anniversary - so there was plenty of cake to go round.

Speeches during the break for food were emotional where Karl, my father-in-law and I all stood up to share emotional words. Following this, Karl and I danced to 'Up Where we Belong'[1]. This was the song we had chosen for our first dance at our wedding 17 years earlier. It was very special to us, and we wanted to do it all over again. The lyrics were relevant even more now. We didn't know what tomorrow would bring. We didn't know what adversity would be thrown at us. *There was no time to cry. It's about being alive today, in our NOW moments, lifting us up from the depths of adversity to a clear new perspective, finding all those special moments one after another.* Little did I realise back then, that this wonderful song had so much meaning, especially now at the age of 40! It was so important to dance this dance again! I had even considered wearing my wedding dress to the party, creating a 'fairy godmother' character. My wedding dress would have been ideal, being a 'shell pink' colour. Part of me wished I'd have chosen this outfit now.

Karl and I didn't know what lay ahead that week and we wanted this to be a very special memory. The evening was just wonderful. We had so much fun that night. As everyone left, they wished me all the very best for Tuesday and asked me to let them know. We were absolutely worn out the next day - but it was worth every minute!

On **Tuesday 21st September**, we arrived at 'Georgina Unit' for my appointment with my oncologist. Everyone was on tender hooks. Blood tests, scans and relevant tests had all been completed in the weeks preceding my appointment. Even the nurses were on tender hooks as we arrived. I remember sitting in the reception area opposite the receptionist's desk, just waiting quietly, watching what was going on around me, thinking ... *'Has all this really happened to me? Have I really got to the end of my treatment? I've been coming here for 6 months now. I'm sure I will be ok, 'it's OK', I feel ok.'*

Next thing I know ... *"Michelle Townsend?"* A nurse called my name.

"Yes, that's me." Both Karl and I stood up, entering the room where my oncologist doctor was sitting waiting for us.

"How are we doing Michelle? Good to see you today," was his greeting.

"I'm good thank you. We are good."

He then went on to say ... *"I have just been looking through your reports and results from the last tests you've received. I'm pleased to say that your treatment has been successful. We are very pleased with how you have responded."*

It was like the words flowed out of his mouth in slow motion. Both Karl and I released a big sigh of relief in unison. A great big smile appeared across my face and the relief on both of our faces just said it all. You could see the emotions flowing within our eyes. Karl burst into tears of joy and relief.

"I did it! That's the news I wanted to hear! Thank you so so much!"

"You have been incredibly positive throughout your treatment Michelle; it's been good to see. I just need to go through a few things with you and then we can let you go. Hodgkin's Lymphoma creates changes in the blood that cannot be reversed. Therefore, you will be required to carry an NHS card warning that you are at risk of 'transfusion - associated graft - versus - host disease'."

"That sounds technical!" I said, as he filled in the card with my details.

"You'll need to carry this card with you for the rest of your life just in case you ever required a blood transfusion. Cellular blood components (Red cells and platelets) must be GAMMA IRRADIATED, otherwise a cytokine storm can take place and can be life threatening."

"Right, ok. Thank you." It all sounded fascinating and something I would research more in the following weeks to understand more.

Dates were put in place for my follow-on check-ups. We thanked the doctor and nurse and left the room stepping into the next part of this journey. As we stepped back into the reception area, all the nurses cheered and congratulated me on the news of my positive results. I was then signed out from being an in-patient to an out-patient. As we said our thank yous and goodbyes, we walked out of the hospital feeling at peace. It's done! It's over!

Back home, everyone was waiting patiently to hear my results. Needless to say, everyone was over the moon and so relieved. When Aaron and Ethan returned home from school, I welcomed them with an almighty hug telling them the news.

They were so happy. Although I don't think at their ages they would ever have realised the depths of what had gone on over the last 6 months.

In the months that followed, regular trips back to the hospital resumed. Initially every 6 months, changing to 12 months. It was very weird not going on a regular basis. During treatment, there seemed a sense of security there. Now the visits had stopped, the only way I could describe it was - I was missing going, missing the routine, I felt a bit lost and didn't have the reassurance that treatment was keeping cancer away. Deep down, I knew my positive mindset was working brilliantly. I trusted everything was going to be OK, *it's OK'*, but slowly I went downhill and by March 2011, I was low. I had built up this approach that ... *'When I've finished treatment, we will do this - when I've finished treatment, we will do that.'* I was going to do lots of different things. Life looked completely different on the 'other side', but in the end it wasn't. It almost felt like a let-down. Not wanting to sound ungrateful here, but it's how I felt. I don't know what I was expecting really. This put a lot of pressure on Karl. Eventually, I adjusted back into normal life and slowly the memories started to fade into the distance. Cancer wasn't thought about much, learning how to live again from a new perspective, knowing I had been given a second chance. We started cruising, going to Norway for Karl's 40th birthday, making a point of making special memories, enjoying the children growing up. I continued with my mind work, knowing my thoughts can create my reality.

'Georgina Unit' had helped so much, so in 2013 I decided to organise two music concerts for my pupils to raise money for 'The Leukaemia Unit Appeal Fund' who support the Unit. They were a great success! All pupils did me proud; they enjoyed learning and performing their chosen pieces, knowing they were doing something positive for charity. The concerts raised a grand total of £2600 for the Unit. The money helped towards the new pod - a waiting area which was being built at Russells Hall Hospital.

My 2014 appointment came as a lovely surprise.

"We are so pleased with you Michelle that we are going to discharge you today. We no longer require you to come back for your check-ups, you are free to go!"

Those were the best words we could have heard. As we stepped out of the hospital, I felt as free as a butterfly. I had been in my chrysalis for too long now. I'd learnt a lot in that cocoon. Now, I was allowed to fly into *'freedom'*. In June 2014, I really honoured that freedom by buying a new car which we saw as we casually walked round a garage. I'd always wanted a convertible and there in front of me was a metallic dark purple Fiat 500C with 7 miles on the clock. So, I bought it there and then! I thought ... *'Why not? Life is for living.'* I've always loved and been proud of my cars and it felt good to be back in the driving seat of life, so to speak.

WOW! Within 4 years, I was discharged. Life was looking good, except in the months and years that followed - Karl kept going on about the survival outcome of reaching 2 years, 5 years, 10 years past treatment and I couldn't deal with it. It was bothering me. Every time he mentioned it, I felt on borrowed time. My approach was that I was living life - no matter what. It didn't matter how many years I had left. I was alive and living. I didn't want to focus on the likelihood of making it to a certain date or not. It wasn't necessary or an option. Karl was trying to use it as reassurance - I understood that, but we didn't need to focus there at all. Then, in 2014, our relationship started to change. I was falling out of love with him. He seemed more like a brother to me than my husband. It was Karl's turn to venture into a downhill slope, eventually hitting rock bottom.

"I have had enough of this reaching 2 years, 5 years, thing, I can't do this anymore. You either change and we start living what life I have left, or I'm done! I haven't gone through all this pain and adversity to keep going down the 'what if' route. I've done it to live! To enjoy life, no matter how long I have left!" I was stern, something I didn't usually do with Karl, but I'd had enough. I couldn't do it anymore. It was a wake-up call for Karl. We both had to change our perspective, otherwise our relationship wasn't going to survive.

I can see now that I didn't realise how bad things had got for Karl. He'd had some help in the early stages of my illness from the Hospital councillor, McMillan, and our GP Surgery. All of which let him down. This resulted in a telephone consultation and a questionnaire which ended up leaving him in a very dark place - it made things worse. Finally, after seeing a different GP who was supportive on a regular basis, Karl ended up on anti-depressants, which allowed him space to sort his head out. I was frustrated at this time because all of this didn't fit with my thought processes and how I had dealt with the situation. Because of this, we lost communication with each other. Karl became lost and his self-esteem and confidence vanished.

Eventually it peaked and he said he was leaving. I didn't want this. I wanted the relationship to work. I wanted us to work - we were good together. We always knew what each other was doing without speaking a word. We communicated without speaking. We knew each other so well. I didn't allow him to go, but made it quite clear that we had to focus past cancer now and let it go completely. There was no point in holding onto it any longer. If I could let it go, Karl could too. I know his response was because he was so worried about losing me. He was living in a dreadful state of fear, but we couldn't live like that. What was the point? That's not living. That's existing!

Eventually, after resetting and restarting our relationship, things improved wonderfully. We started dating again like a courting couple, changing our approach. Then, finally in

December 2016, we booked a short break to Dublin, where we finally reconnected. We were back on track. We returned on Christmas Eve and never looked back.

A Way Will be Found

Karl and I had a completely different perspective going on in those years. Karl was focused on the physical reality, whereas I was focused on an energetic level, connecting into possibilities that I could not yet see, the mind/body connection. I was trusting that everything was OK, already sorted. Karl couldn't get to that place, believing only in what he saw in front of him. Focusing my mind where I wanted to be came from my experience with EHS. This wasn't something new for me. I'd applied it for many years, I'd had plenty of practice, now applying it to the cancer journey. I trusted it. The shift in consciousness pulled us apart; we weren't resonating on the same wavelength. Karl in the frequency of *'fear'*, me in the frequency of *'freedom'*. I had already moved *'from fear to freedom'* processing EHS. I remained in the *'freedom'* state to help me through cancer. Karl was now learning to trust that things can change and that ... *'it's OK'* - creating positive change in the way that felt right for him.

There are many fantastic techniques out there which can be used to help refocus us, bringing in a new perspective. Worrying about whether techniques are being done correctly is usually what puts blocks in place and stops us from using them. Taking the techniques and developing them into your own style works wonders. We are all different - no two people are the same - everyone has different life experiences. Applying a different approach or a slight twist can bring life-changing results - perceiving with your own eyes and adjusting so that the technique works for you in the best possible way. Techniques, rules and guidance have all been created or invented in the first place by a person. Someone had to think about these techniques, write them down and develop them. When we adapt these techniques to our own personal comfort zone, they are less likely to be discarded; thus, we utilise them on a more continuous basis because it suits us as a person. Karl and I had been the perfect example of adapting.

The wonderful 'OK *technique*', which I have shared with many of my clients, has slowly evolved over the years. I just chose to use the word 'OK', as it fitted with me. I had a habit of saying 'OK' when I presented my music concerts - always chuckling about it - so 'OK' seemed relevant to use. It was important to work with and choose a technique that resonated with me. I could access 'OK' quickly, addressing situations in any moment. It became the most powerful technique I ever used. 'OK' allowed me to make friends with the situation, address and question the *'energy'*, thus allowing me to let go and sending it on with love. EHS had already proved that getting into an argument with situations fires up and adds to the *'energy'* around it, feeding it and making it stronger - feeding the *'fear'* and bringing it more into focus. Thus, making it more likely to come firing right back in your face!

This wonderful *'OK'* technique I'm talking about may seem a little bizarre, strange to some, but it works extremely well with an open mind. Remembering that feelings are usually the first indication of a response, followed by thoughts, we can create change in any moment - and very quickly - using a word and an action.

'OK Technique' (Left to Right Technique)

- *'Awareness'* – Become aware of the initial feeling, thought or response.
- *'Acknowledgement'* – Imagine the situation at hand external to you. See the situation/thought/worry to the left-hand side of you, as if it's a person or bubble of energy.

- *'Acceptance'* – Speak to the situation/thought/worry like a person, your best friend. Don't turn it away or get angry with it. Accept it is there.

- *'Address'* – Address it with … "OK' I am aware that you are there. Thank you for reminding me.' This allows you to perceive the situation/thought/worry external to you, from a different perspective, stepping back from it, so to speak.

- *'Refocus'* – 'Thank you for reminding me that I can use this situation/thought/worry as a direction for change, considering a new response and new outlook, thus bringing in the new perspective.'

- *'Choice'* – 'I am aware that you (*'you'* because you are talking to that part of 'you' to the left) have been responding this way, but I am now choosing to focus over here.'

- *'New Direction'* – Redirect to the right-hand side of you with new perspective.

This may seem long winded, but it isn't. It can be done in a split second. Let me give you an example of how to address an anxiety response to make it easier to understand. Remember the *'you (anxious)'* is the anxious part of you that you have removed to have a chat with. *'I'* is you talking to *'you'* the anxious part of you.

'OK', *'I'* have become aware of feeling anxious (**Awareness** and **Acknowledgement.** See 'anxious you' on your left-hand side).

'OK', *'I'* accept this is how *'you (anxious)'* feel right now (**Acceptance**).

'OK', *'I'* am aware that *'you (anxious)'* are there, thank *'you (anxious)'* for reminding me of this response (**Address**).

'OK', *'we ('you' and 'I' together)'* can use this feeling of adversity to create the change. Consider the new perspective option. (**Refocus**).

'OK', *'you (anxious)'* know you have a choice in any moment of how to respond - YES.

'You (anxious)' understand that all this has come from old thoughts and experiences which are in the past - YES.

Do *'you (anxious)'* need to hold onto the past? - NO.

Are *'you (anxious)'* going to allow this feeling to affect our future? - NO.

The past can't be changed, but *'you (anxious)'* know you can affect the future by thinking and responding differently right NOW! - YES.

This response does not benefit *'us ('you' and 'I' together)',* so are *'you (anxious)'* willing to come over here with *'me (I)'* in this new choice of thought and response? - YES.

All the worry in the world won't change this anxiousness - I KNOW.

This anxiousness is being created by *'you (anxious)'* through your thoughts - YES.

You have the power to change this right NOW! - YES. (**Choice**).

'OK', let's look at this anxiousness this way over here (see the new perspective on right-hand side of you).

We *('you' and 'I' together)* can create an understanding that we see things more clearly from a place of calm. Even though this is an anxious time, we can choose to see it from a new place, considering different approaches. Adversity strengthens us, so why don't we venture over here to the right and use it to empower us from this moment? (**Refocus – New Perspective**).

This 'OK' technique can be utilised with any thought or response you wish to change. Experiment with it, play around with it, make it your own. Remembering that a thought or response can be addressed within seconds. You are only one thought away from calmness and one thought away from anxiousness. It's your choice!

References:

[1] Nitzsche, J., Sainte-Marie, B., & Jennings, W. (1982). *Up Where We Belong.* [Recorded by] Cocker, J., & Warnes, J. On *An Officer and a Gentleman.* [Medium of recording]. Island

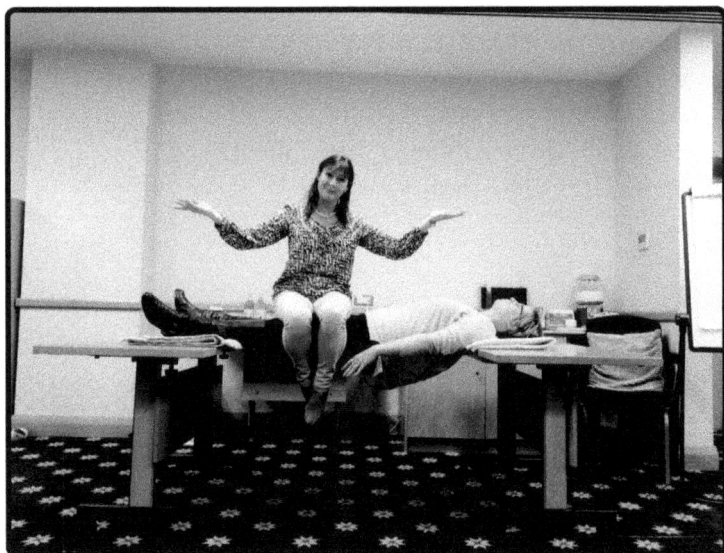

The' Rod of Iron' exercise, with Jacqueline sitting on my middle, showing the power of hypnosis, October 2015.

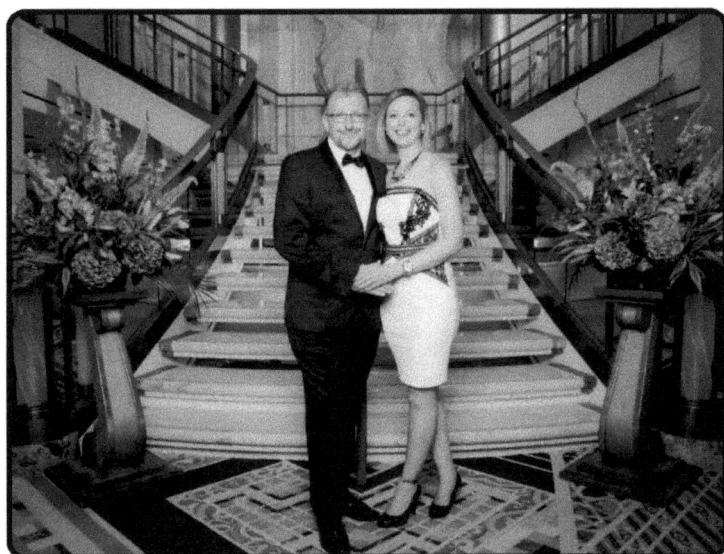

Me, with Karl on our P&O Aurora
cruising holiday, August 2019.

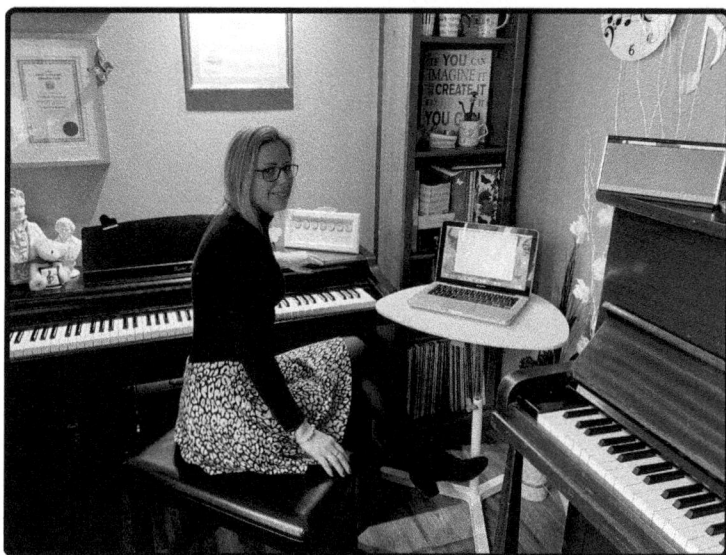

Learning to 'Zoom in'. Teaching online
during Covid, March 2020.

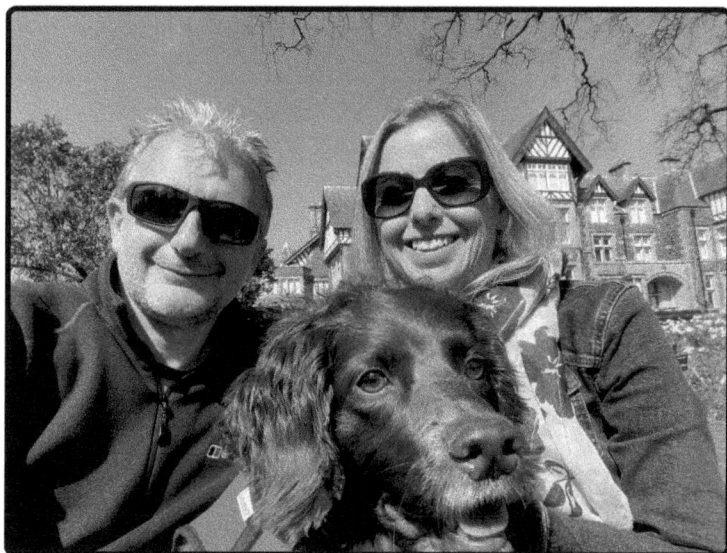

Our beautiful Tess during a day out to Bodnant
Gardens, Wales, April 2021.

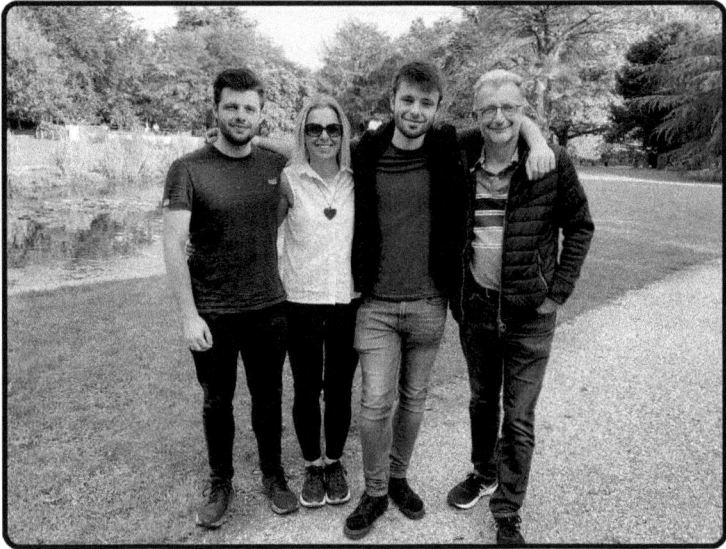

Family photo time in London, October 2021.

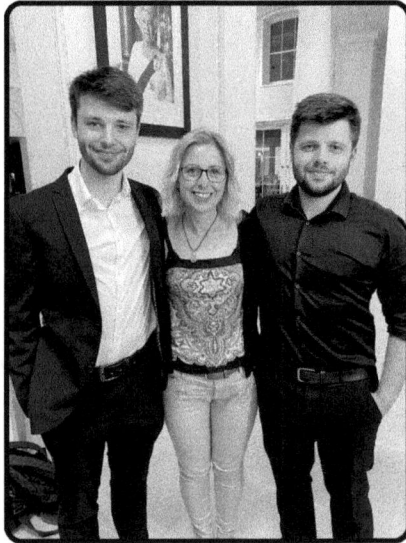

Me, with Aaron and Ethan at Aaron's final
recital at Royal College of Music, May 2022.

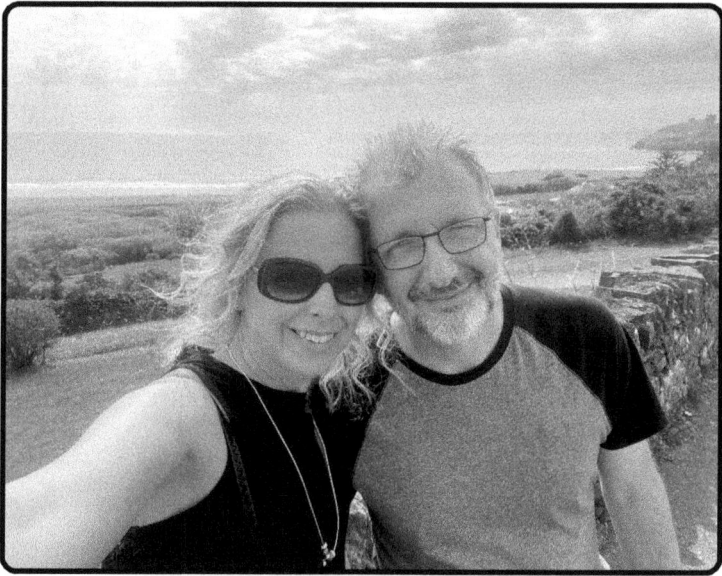

Me, with Karl in North Wales, April 2023.

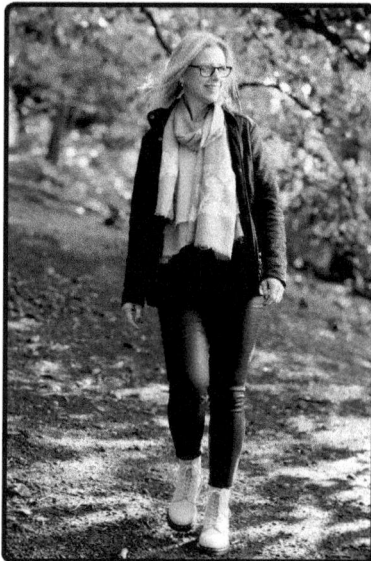

Connecting with nature on my professional photo shoot
at Himley Hall, September 2023.

Michelle Townsend

Part III

Therapies to Therapist

Chapter 17

Time for a Change

'When you feel lost, you are in fact finding yourself. The uncomfortable feeling pushes you to search, pushes you to find something new, pushes you to visualise different options. Rather than thinking you are lost, connect with the feeling of creation; then flow with the new 'energy' that comes forth.'

~ Michelle Townsend

I'd recovered from EHS. I'd recovered from Hodgkin's Lymphoma Cancer. Life was good. I felt blessed I'd been allowed to live, or should I say, 'allowed' myself to live. But deep down I was totally lost - something was missing. It was like I was out in the Sahara Desert, walking constantly, looking for the water hole to drink. I kept seeing the oases, but they weren't really there. What was going on? Why was I feeling like this? Why would I feel like this. Especially after recovering from such adverse experiences? I was extremely lucky!! Lucky to be alive for heaven's sake! I *should* be happy and content. Although, those *'shoulds'* of being happy, weren't necessarily what *should* happen if I was not allowing my true path of life to flow. It was depressing me. Bringing me down. I felt I had no sense of direction in my life anymore and I was just ticking over doing the same old, same old. Just existing. I knew it was down to me to make the right decisions in life for myself, but sometimes, do we really know what we want? We've all been there. I wanted and needed something new - a new focus - something to kick my brain into gear; to feel the ecstatic feelings of excitement again. I just didn't know what. I loved my music and my teaching. That side of my career, running my music business was doing amazing. It always had flowed, but it wasn't enough anymore. I felt I had more to give to life; there was something else there waiting to blossom. I felt as though I was here in this life to do more. I was being guided, drawn. I'd been given a second chance. This new sense of direction just felt blocked because I really didn't know what I wanted.

One afternoon, I was sitting in our conservatory, feeling like a rabbit in the headlights not knowing which way to turn. I felt a sense of panic come over me. I didn't know what to do or where to put myself.

"I need to do something new, something different, but I don't know what." I suddenly said to Karl.

He seemed quite shocked, but was also aware that I hadn't been myself for some time.

"Have a look on the college website to give you some ideas, maybe that will help guide you. What about something holistic? Maybe hairdressing or massage." He responded.

I'd always wanted to do hairdressing at one stage. I'd make a good hairdresser. I realised this during covid, in 2020. I became the household hairdresser - and a good one at that - I must say!

The holistic side especially fascinated me. I was looking at massage, Indian head massage, Reiki, all these types of subjects. I had even considered training to become a yoga teacher before now. This was how I came to find my amazing Yoga Teacher, Anne Griffiths - I still attend her wonderful, mindful, relaxing 'YogaBubble'[1] classes now. The only problem with all the courses I was considering was they were all evening classes. I worked evenings teaching piano. Everything I was considering was being blocked - my music teaching was stopping me! I became more and more frustrated and upset. I just wanted this feeling of frustration - this lost feeling to go away. I needed new direction.

I have come to learn from my journey that we *do* put our own blocks in place. '*We create our own reality*' - whether we believe we do or not. I accept full responsibility for the EHS and cancer I experienced. My friends and family may disagree, but I can see it as clear as day. Nothing comes into our experience unless we activate that frequency within us - whether it's something wanted or not - it's a hard pill to swallow. Emotions run at a deep subconscious level from the programs we run. We are just a walking set of programs running our 'app'!

When pushing so hard, wanting something to fall into place, blocks can appear, preventing that something coming into our experience, into existence. This is why people find healing or recovery hard. The sheer wanting and desperation sends out the message of not having it, thus emitting the wrong '*energy*' - the '*energy*' of where we are, without it. Why do we do this? **We** become too focused on reality and ego! What we should be remembering, is the subconscious only works with NOW - it doesn't understand the difference between reality or whether we are imaging/thinking it. Project that '*trust, faith and belief*', visualise a foregone conclusion - seeing through the reality so to speak, just like I did. Situations, scenarios and reality can then start to change. The body responds to the mind. Our actions will then follow to create that reality. It must be. It's physics, quantum physics, the universe - 'we get what we focus on' remember!

My understanding about '*frequency*' and '*energy*' is reflected in many ways throughout my book. We are all electromagnetic beings giving off the frequency of how we are feeling via our emotions. The frequency I was emitting in Summer 2015 was frustration and feeling lost. Why would anything show up to guide me? Except send more frequency to be frustrated about! It's obvious that only things would match that frustration frequency. It's only when I changed my focus and perception that I allowed things to fall into place - where I could bring what I was wanting into my experience.

So ... things were about to get interesting. I was about to be reminded just how powerful the *'law of attraction'* was yet again.

In all the frustration, I decided to step back from pushing too hard to find something new. I handed it over to the universe.

'Something will come up; give me the prompt, the guidance I need' I said. I just let it go that afternoon after discussing it briefly with Karl.

To my surprise, I started to notice I was thinking more clearly. Well, I shouldn't say surprise really, because I know all this. I know how a change of focus and change of *'energy'* works. *'Acceptance'* is the key to letting go after all. Having played about with this over the years, I often chuckle to myself. When I went through my chemotherapy treatment, I just let things go, accepted - everything flowed easily, everything fell into place. I didn't put any effort into making things happen back then. I never forced anything - I just had that *'trust, faith and belief'* in place. I remained calm throughout the experience. Things were about to fall into place once again.

I suddenly had the thought, urge and realisation ... *'Why don't I train to become a hypnotherapist? I'd love to do what Mike does.'* Ever since I'd received my first few hypnotherapy sessions with Mike, I'd thought how amazing it was to be able to help people in that way. It was extremely powerful. After all I had been through - everything I had learnt about the mind - every positive response I had experienced from having hypnotherapy sessions, I thought … *'I could do this! I could help people; help people with cancer and Electromagnetic Hypersensitivity … I could do this!'* I kept repeating this over and over in my mind. Imagine what I could do from these adverse experiences I had overcome, what I could share with people. My actions took over and I started to flow. I was finally in gear!

At that moment, I had the urge to ring Mike to see if he knew where I could get hypnotherapy training from. I really hoped he was free to talk. I dialled his number … he answered … *'Great!'* He instantly recommended his friend Jacqueline who lived in South London.

"I'm not sure Jacqueline is running a course right now, but give her a call to see if she is planning one soon. You've nothing to lose. I know she hasn't run one recently, but you never know, it's worth contacting her," he said.

Mike thought it was a great idea. *"You'll make a good therapist Michelle, after what you've overcome and changed in your own life."*

I felt so excited, I felt like I'd found that something new. So … I followed the feeling, let the actions come forward, let them continue to flow. After coming off the phone to Mike, I spoke with Karl regarding my thoughts.

Karl said … *"If that's what you really feel you want to do, we will find a way for you to do it."*

Money was a bit tight at this time, but Karl reassured me we would find a way for me to do this. I would, of course, have to travel to South London, which would incur costs on top of the course. However, I just followed the feeling and continued my actions of creating my next steps. I knew everything would all fall into place.

I rang Jacqueline that afternoon. Once again, to my surprise she answered. Everything was just falling into place extremely quickly. I explained I was Mike's friend and about my current feelings of wanting to do something new after the journey I had gone through. We had a lovely conversation. I felt really at ease talking to Jacqueline.

When I asked the question ... *"Are you running a Hypnotherapy Training Course soon?"*

Jacqueline replied ... *"Well actually, yes, I am, Michelle. I've had a break for a while, but I have one starting in October. There is a pre-requisite to attend the Self-Hypnosis Course first; this will be in October. The main training then starts shortly after that."*

I remember standing in our bedroom having the conversation with a great big grin on my face. I just knew this was the right direction for me, I just had to go for it. Everything was flowing to make this happen. I couldn't believe how quickly everything was taking shape. After we finished our conversation, Jacqueline said she would send me an email with all the details and information regarding the course and dates. She told me to have a good look through, and check to see if all were suitable, then let her know if I was willing and happy to go ahead. I agreed. I came off the phone feeling ecstatic! I felt like a big weight had been lifted. My *'energy'* was now flowing again. I had obviously released the frustration - I now had a purpose, a direction again. Possibilities had opened up for me in a matter of hours ... *'Oh wow!'* When situations fall into place, the universe positions, aligns and allows it to happen. As the saying goes ... *'It only takes one **yes** for things to fall into place'.*

A Way Will Be Found

The *'law of attraction'* strikes again! This time it was a very powerful reminder that 'LOA' does absolutely work! Focus - get to the feeling place - trust - then allow. Frequencies always match.

Sometimes, we need reminders, to kick us up the butt! Giving us a shake-up. Losing our sense of direction can in fact be good for us. It opens portals within our mind which give us guided direction - striving to look for answers, a new focus where we wouldn't have looked before. We realise how far we have come, what we have learnt - we are then drawn to expand on that knowledge and develop it further.

It was highlighted to me again that I did 'create my own reality'. I was in control at every point. Even though I felt out of control at that moment in the conservatory - that was the guidance coming through. If I had not have experienced the feeling of frustration, it would not have driven me to look - to search - to find that something new. It would not have been on my radar. Needing a new focus was a must at this point in my life. It was creating purpose - I had now found that 'human need' that I had been missing!

References:

1. Griffiths, A. *YogaBubble*. https://www.yogabubble.net

Michelle Townsend

Chapter 18

Rod of Iron

*'You are like a rod of iron! You conduct electrical energy.
You magnetise like a lightning strike. You are strong, secure
and resilient.'*

*'As you attract different situations in your life, remember ...
stand in your own power and strength!'*

~ Michelle Townsend

In **October 2015**, after my feelings of being lost and in turmoil, I was now booked on 'The College of Inspirational Hypnotherapy' Diploma in Hypnotherapy and Psychotherapy Course, with Jacqueline Panchaud as my trainer. To say I was so excited about this new venture was an understatement! I needed to do something else with my life. I now had a strong sense of direction. The feeling of being lost had now dissipated.

The pre-requisite for the course was a weekend of self-hypnosis training. I knew this would allow me to help others navigate their life's journeys too, no matter what was being thrown at them. My life experiences so far had certainly been a powerful teaching to me - I had after all just come through a cancer journey. I had used hypnotherapy to create powerful change in my life. It would allow me to utilise all the knowledge I had accumulated from that sheer adversity ... and why not use it? Adding 'hypnotherapy' to my CV would be an amazing achievement! It felt right. I felt comfortable with my decision.

The Self-Hypnosis Course was at a conference hall at the Business Centre, Hilton London, Gatwick. I knew how powerful hypnosis was. Learning more about self-hypnosis was important to me. Little did I realise just how much. I had already been using self-hypnosis from hypnotherapy sessions with Mike. What I didn't realise was how amazing this weekend was going to be in developing my knowledge further.

This journey was proving to be very special - it was also pushing me to venture into things I had never done before. I was certainly being put into the *'feel the fear and do it anyway'*[1] situation! Having never travelled too far on motorways driving alone before, I asked Karl if he would accompany me - making a weekend of it. Whilst I was on the course, Karl ventured off in the local area. The journey also acted as a pre-run for me driving alone to attend my hypnotherapy training in the months that followed. It felt exciting, but nerve-racking! 170 miles nerve racking! Making this decision to train in hypnotherapy had pushed me into new experiences which felt inspiring.

Attempting new things pushes us into situations that initially may feel uncomfortable. On the other hand, it also leads us to new places, new people, new situations and life experiences. As life has gone on, I have come to realise leading a sheltered life doesn't really do you much good. Working from home had created that isolation, even having clients attending for music lessons or hypnotherapy sessions. I love my jobs and the communications it creates and brings for me, but even now I still find it lonely working from home. It's important to be out there, doing those new things, experiencing life and the social aspect that can project us forward in ways we never thought possible. Stepping forward makes us realise just how strong we actually are. Things are possible - anything is possible if we put our mind to it - navigating most things and achieving more than we could ever realise. It's just taking the first step. We don't know until we do it! We are like a *'rod of iron'* more than we realise - strong, safe and secure. We find every bit of that strength when needed. This new course and direction reaffirmed that to me. I was about to learn a lot. My perspective was about to be changed yet again!

Saturday 10th October 2015

Karl and I had a lovely trip to Gatwick early that morning, arriving at around 9.30am, where I got chatting to other attendees. Looking back now, a lot of the people who attended this weekend course were on the Hypnotherapy Diploma Course in the months that followed. Some were doing refresher courses. It was lovely bringing us all together.

Following a fascinating day of listening to Jacqueline, completing exercises and learning plenty of new knowledge, Karl came to pick me up. We then ventured off for a lovely evening at our hotel.

Sunday 11th October 2015

The knowledge continued, learning about the mind and its different aspects throughout the day. We had now also learnt how to put ourselves into hypnosis - the course took this to an even deeper level for me. There's always room for more knowledge - we never stop learning.

Towards the end of the course, Jacqueline, our trainer did an exercise that would show the power of the subconscious mind, taking it to the limit of understanding. First, the group were shown some photos of previous weekend courses where people had done these exercises. One such exercise was the *'Rod of Iron'* as I nicknamed it. You could see clearly on the photos people supported between two tables, high off the floor.

To add to this, you could also see an adult sitting on top of them! Looking at these photos it seemed unreal. How on earth would, or could this be possible? How can an adult support themselves between two tables just on their own to start with - let alone with an adult sitting on their middle? It was unbelievable, but happening in the photo.

Each of us took it in turns to do this exercise. I watched with amazement! Lying on the floor, we each put ourselves into hypnosis as Jacqueline had taught us. She then guided us, directing parts of our body to be as strong as a *'rod of iron'* - strong, safe and secure. Each time she asked us a question, we visualized that process taking place within our body. We agreed on each step of the way when we felt it had taken place.

I was third to do the exercise. As I put myself into hypnosis, I realised my heart was beating very fast, feeling concerned people could see the pulse in my neck. I have always had a strong, fast heartbeat and it was certainly beating fast at this moment! I really didn't feel calm and relaxed at all. Thoughts were going through my head ... *'How on earth was I going to put myself in hypnosis feeling like this? I'm not relaxed! How could this be possible?'* There was almost an element of conscious doubt. I felt like I was too conscious, working more with the conscious mind rather than the subconscious. *'Surely, I will collapse between the tables?'* After instructions from Jacqueline, other people in the class helped to pick my body up off the floor and place me between the tables - my head resting on one table, my feet by my ankles resting on the other. Nothing else was in-between - I was floating supported between two tables... WOW! I was even fully aware of this! *'Am I really in hypnosis here? I must be?'*

After a couple of minutes, Jacqueline said ... *"Right - let's see how strong this body of iron is, this body of Michelle's, which is like a rod of iron."*

Jacqueline made me aware she was going to climb on top of the middle area of my body. She climbed on from the side where my legs were positioned on the table. She then shuffled herself across to my middle. To my surprise, she then bounced slightly, showing how strong I was. I had an adult sitting on top of me with no support underneath, hovering a good metre above the floor! If I had collapsed, I would have done some serious damage to my back and spine, but I remained a *'rod of iron'*.

Jacqueline climbed off me; my fellow course friends then lifted me off the tables placing me back on the floor, where I brought myself out of hypnosis. I sat up and started to fill up with tears because since having chemotherapy, my strength was not brilliant. I felt that my limbs were much weaker, no longer a strong person. This exercise had proved to me that we can change our thoughts and responses in an instant, creating powerful change in our body in that moment. If I could do what I had just done, what else could I achieve? It was extremely powerful. It also proved the subconscious works with NOW!

***

Because of the many trips I was about to embark on travelling to South London for my hypnotherapy training, I chose to do a powerful hypnosis session on myself. I put the amazing knowledge and reassurance I'd gained from the self-hypnosis weekend into use - here's why ......

I'd had many wonderful mini cruises with my sister. During a return trip home from Southampton whilst travelling along the M27 motorway, I was aware that I was tired, so we pulled over for a coffee. It's always wise if feeling that way. Back on the motorway, I still felt tired and thought ... *'I'll be ok, I'll stay awake'.* Next thing I knew, I was hearing horns sounding from a lorry behind me. I suddenly realised the lorry driver was flashing his lights and I could see a white car to the right-hand side of me rather close.

To add to this, my sister was shouting ... *"Shell!"* ... and reaching to grab the steering wheel.

I realised in that split second, I'd fallen asleep at the wheel! My sister had also closed her eyes. The lorry driver had done his job in alerting us both and a good job at that! I was just a couple of feet away from the side of the white car and I'd veered over the white lines on the road. The road was also turning to the left, so I would have gone further over in just a second longer. OH MY GOD! My heart was pounding, I started to shake and felt panic set in.

Emma, my sister, calmed me down ... *"It's ok, nothing happened, we are safe."*

But I kept thinking of what could have happened. It freaked me out completely, thinking I could have killed us both and someone else. It still makes me feel uncomfortable to this day. I can't really talk about it. Whilst writing this, my heart was pounding and a feeling of dread took over me (subconscious responses from memories). Next chance we got, we pulled over. I needed to calm down. The shock was rippling through every part of my body - it was this that kept both of us awake for the rest of the journey home.

... The hypnosis session was to keep me awake as soon as I saw white lines on any motorway or dual carriageway. I spent a good hour visualising being awake ... *'Whilst driving each and every inch of the motorway, I remain alert, awake, and find the journey an enjoyable experience. Seeing the white lines keeps me alert every inch of the way,'* was my affirmation. It sorted it! I've had no problems since, apart from a short spell of where I fell asleep as passenger whilst Karl was driving. I would suddenly become alert and then go to grab the steering wheel. Obviously, this became a problem, as it was making Karl jump, which could also have caused issues. I'd only done the original hypnosis as a driver and not as passenger - the subconscious listens very carefully; it's specific. So, once again another hypnosis session -

this time as a passenger and it was all sorted! It's very powerful! My subconscious just wanted to do its best for me. Protect me from what it believed to be true. So it did! My subconscious was creating responses from the experience, the memory. This needed to be changed and new responses created. I guided 'subby' with the outcome and used adversity to create change.

***

As I arrived at the venue to start my training to become a hypnotherapist, I could see familiar faces. There were 10 people on the course - most of them knew each other. Living down South, their journeys were easier and shorter than mine. I had to travel from the Midlands every month, which was a jaunt, but worth it and I did it! It was another experience that increased my confidence in driving all that way on my own. Most of the time Karl came with me, but the first few journeys I did by myself. Even driving back in thick fog! I was very proud of myself. I had never driven that far on my own, apart from driving to Southampton with my sister for our mini cruises. There were a lot of things I did that initially seemed very daunting, but I got through them every time.

On attending the first training session, I felt quite nervous not really knowing anyone. Which I suppose is acceptable? I just wish I could be myself initially, feel more confident and not shy, although, this is something that has improved over time. Running my groups, meeting clients and running hypnotherapy sessions has helped resolve this.

I remember our second training day. We had to do a hypnotherapy induction on one of our fellow students. It was so nerve racking. *'How the hell am I going to do this? Can I actually become a hypnotherapist?'* Again, I had all sorts going through my head. It almost seemed impossible. Though, like anything else before, I got through it. Each time we practised taking each other into hypnosis, it got easier and easier, adding more steps along the way. With the knowledge Jacqueline was sharing, I kept thinking ... *'How do I do this? How will I know what to do in any hypnotherapy session?'* But when I seemed to have a mental block - the right thing always came to me. The worry always was ... *'Am I good enough to do this?'* Well ... yes ... I am! I always know what to use, I'm always guided. Jacqueline taught us the tools to have in our therapy bag. Thankfully, we were taught non-script hypnotherapy - which means sessions are adapted for each client, making it a more personal journey for them, thus more likely to be successful. Each person is different and has different experiences.

I qualified as a hypnotherapist on 12th June 2016, passing with flying colours! The training from Jacqueline Panchaud had been so fascinating and inspirational. I am truly thankful for all the knowledge she shared. It felt amazing that I could now put everything I had learnt into use, including my knowledge from my own adversities and experiences. I knew it would help so many. By the end of 2016, my life was about to change yet again. What this course had highlighted to me was to trust myself, that I can do anything I put my mind to, no matter how difficult it may seem. Where does anyone start? At the beginning! It takes practice to get better at something - practice and making the effort!

A Way Will Be Found

I used 'self-hypnosis' on a regular basis during my EHS journey and chemotherapy treatment. Often just allowing myself time out from thoughts. I wasn't particularly directing a specific focus. I just found it helpful to just BE. Other times I would go inwardly to visualise - sending in what I call 'my little men' to the area that needed help, whether it be thoughts, a part of my body, or my cells. Wearing their white hard hats with big red crosses on the front, 'my little men' would get on with helping and healing. The subconscious takes this on board.

I can't reiterate enough, that when we have a good understanding of how our mind works, we have the power to create change in our lives.

From my journey through dis-ease, I've ventured down many paths, used various techniques and applied various thought processes to create change. Life continues to be a wonderful journey of enlightenment - always learning. Especially during my training. Believe me, I've tested them! As a therapist, I can utilise these techniques with clients, and of course continuing to use them for myself as and when necessary. I have come to trust the techniques; I have *faith and belief* in them. Working on myself for many years, I have found there is a tendency to focus on a specific technique at any one time - that's what I've experienced along my journey. There are many techniques to utilise, but I find I stick with one or two specific ones. Using the one that resonates for that moment. As I have become aware of a new technique, I tend to get a little excited about using it, focused on applying it. It's a new focus. New things feel good, creating a clear perspective. Having something new creates fascination, becoming drawn in, intrigued to see if it's going to work. It's almost like a new adventure.

I was coming to understand these techniques more as I developed further along my hypnotherapy training, especially being trained as a non-script therapist. Personalising the therapy for each client helps adapt the techniques for yourself too. I had been doing this for years on my healing journey without even realising! The bonus is, there are many at hand, in the toolbox, when needed. It's reassuring that they are there to literally grab hold of at times of change, or when you want to make a change in your life. Thinking of them as a tool in our 'mental toolbox' gives us choice, freedom and guidance at any point in time.

Our toolbox for life is constantly being updated and added to as we travel on our own journeys and experiences. Our subconscious logs away information from our experiences. It also adds our perceptions and feelings related to those experiences. Perception is 'Reality'. Our perception can be changed at any time, especially if it doesn't feel right. That's the benefit of having a 'mental toolbox'. Only allowing in the beneficial options that work, dis-guarding what doesn't work. It's refining your first aid for the mind box!

Developing and improving my training of 'self-hypnosis' was proving very powerful and one I now share with many of my clients once they have addressed and made positive changes from their sessions. It's giving them that special space to connect 'in' with their subconscious, where they can go inward to make adjustments themselves. This helps to maintain a healthy thought process, positive outlook and positive responses. It's also about being kind to you. Using 'affirmations', or as I prefer to say 'positive statements' alongside self-hypnosis works extremely well.

A statement to yourself has POWER! Words have POWER! Choose kindness and understanding within. Remember you are always doing your best!

~ Michelle Townsend

It's interesting to think how we talk to ourselves. Imagine if you spoke to your friend in the way you talk inwardly to yourself. How would that make them feel? Would you be boosting that friend with confidence? Or knocking them down in disgust? We are all guilty of knocking ourselves down. Such as … *'I'm no good at that! Why did I say that? I don't have confidence to do that! You are hopeless! I don't like my shape! I could do better! That was totally rubbish!'* We've all done it at some point in our lives - we can be guilty of it daily, beating ourselves up over what we have or haven't done well. I found self-talk so important. I'd ask … *'How do I address myself? Listen to how you talk to yourself?'* Venturing into self-talk was worth it and important. I was pleasantly surprised and shocked at how I did address myself. Most of the time knocking myself down with comments of why I did or didn't do things in a certain way. By starting to address the negative self-talk, things changed. *'You are enough!'* We are always in the right place we need to be. The place we find ourselves in has come from previous thoughts and frequencies which we have given *'energy'* to - so I learnt to say ... *'From this moment forward I give my energy to freedom!'*

Negative situations can be used to create positive situations. Have you ever thought about using a negative to teach learning? We learn more from a negative experience than we do from a positive one. We usually learn not to do it again. People focus on the negative and hold it within them, creating blocks. Why not use the experience and say ... *'Well that didn't go quite as planned, but it has shown me the way to go now. I am now looking at other options that I would have never considered before. If this hadn't have happened, I wouldn't be where I am now'.* That negative experience drives you to a new place of focus that could be life changing, allowing amazing new experiences to come forth into your life. As they say ... *'As one door closes, a new one opens.'* Just imagine learning to look at negatives from that perspective and how your experiences would change! Would you beat yourself up as much? Probably not. You probably wouldn't see it as a negative any longer.

'So ... what is Self-Hypnosis'

It's basically connecting into our 'theta' brain wave patterns. This is where we record and recall our memories. It also connects into the emotional aspect of ourselves. After all, the subconscious is the 'emotional' part of our mind. As with any hypnosis, it is a state of focused attention. Self-hypnosis allows you space. Space to check in with yourself to make positive change and adjustments. A little like doing a guided meditation. A self-hypnosis session could last as long as half an hour, an hour, or even just 1 minute. It all depends on what you want from your personalised session with YOU. We spend most of our lives in hypnosis doing things on autopilot. So, when we choose to direct ourselves specifically into this space, with specific intention, it's amazing what you have access to. You could even call it your 'Control Room'. Clients love that!

It's all about having a clear direction. When working with clients, I direct them through a specific process, training their subconscious to automatically connect quickly and easily to those 'theta' brainwaves. We experience 'theta' brainwaves when we are in a hypnotic state, deep meditation, or light sleep. This also includes REM dream state. Clients gain an in-depth understanding through their sessions, which allows them to utilise self-hypnosis fully. They know what to do. Learning self-hypnosis as part of your hypnotherapy sessions for whatever issue is a common technique therapists share. It's a very good way of maintaining a positive outlook and is extremely good for dealing with anxiety or breaking a habit. It allows you to become self-sufficient at looking after you.

Self-hypnosis can be used for most things. Thoughts, stress, anxiety, illness, pain - both emotional and physical, healing, habits, attracting what you want in life - the list goes on. Most people use it to help stress and anxiety. When we think about stress and anxiety at a deeper level, they are in fact a thought. Thoughts are the root cause creating the response. Stress and anxiety start with a thought. Change the thought and you change the response.

Whether you have done self-hypnosis before or not, let's look at a simplified version. As with all aspects I teach, we want to be keeping it as simple as possible. Why create difficult techniques to dampen your flow?

Beginners' quick Self-Hypnosis Process

The fact that we spend most of our life in hypnosis, we are indeed all able to connect into a hypnotic trance state. It really is just a focused state of attention.

- **GOAL.** Firstly, set your goal of what you are wanting to achieve. Create a positive statement in present tense. E.g. 'I am calm', 'I now experience...'

- **SET INTENTION.** Honour that you are taking time for YOU! Set the intention that you are allowing yourself to connect into your own space. Make sure you are in a safe place, where you feel comfortable.

- **BREATH.** Bring your awareness to your breath. Take three deep breaths in and slowly exhaling out. Allow yourself to settle.

- **CONNECT.** Connect with feeling relaxed. No one can get you while you are here in YOUR space.

- **ADDRESS.** Address any part of you that is experiencing something you want to change or feel uncomfortable with. Check in with YOU. Have a chat to yourself just like you would your best friend. Replace it and focus on the outcome you want, your *goal*.

- **VISUALISE.** Visualise yourself how you want it to be. Remember the subconscious does not distinguish between reality or whether you are imagining/ thinking it. Believing it to be true.

- **POSITIVE STATEMENT.** Spend time visualising, experiencing your goal, repeating your positive statement until you feel you've done enough and feel more comfortable with it. See it in your mind's eye, practise it like it's a foregone conclusion.

- **BREATH.** Focus once again on your breath, start to make gentle movements bringing your awareness to where you are sitting.

- **UP AND OUT.** Count from 1 to 5, making yourself aware you will awaken feeling refreshed, energised and alert as you reach 5. Or simply open your eyes.

This is just a very simple process. It's a basic layout of how to go about self-hypnosis. You don't necessarily have to go 'in' to do any work on yourself. You could just enjoy relaxation and a connection to calm. Take time, as long or short as you need. It really is just a refocus. Enjoy!

References:

1. Jeffers, S. (2007). *Feel The Fear And Do It Anyway*. Vermillion.

Chapter 19

Message from the Other Side

'When we trust our intuition, our gut feeling, the universe responds. It puts situations, blessings and relationships in place, that we would never ever have dreamed of!'

~ Michelle Townsend

October 2016. I had been working voluntary for the 'Georgina Unit Charity Shop' for some time. I felt I was giving a little back for all the help I had received from the 'Georgina Unit' at the hospital during my treatment. Voluntary work is very enriching. It felt good knowing I was offering my time to help others. It's not only beneficial to the people receiving the help, but beneficial for ourselves too. We are giving something back to the community. Giving is receiving - you are emitting the frequency. Kindness is key. When we are kind to others, we are being kind to ourselves also. Kindness boosts oxytocin and dopamine, our feel-good hormones. Being kind also increases serotonin levels. These are neurotransmitters that help regulate our mood. When our mood is regulated, we feel more connected to all around us.

After my hypnotherapy training had finished, I sought ways of developing my new business. Obviously, my music teaching was so important to me. It wasn't even an option to change anything regarding that aspect of my work life. I wanted to find ways of getting out there, sharing my inspirational story to help other cancer sufferers - teaching cancer patients and their families how their mind worked and how it can be used to help in difficult situations such as a cancer journey. White House Cancer Support was a charity where this was a possibility. The funny thing was - a friend had guided me to the White House when I was on my own cancer journey. However, back then it didn't feel right to attend such a place. Yet, here I was now, offering to help and get involved. How bizarre! I rang the White House Cancer Support charity asking if there was anything I could do - to my surprise they suggested running a relaxation group. I started running my group the beginning of November 2016 after ringing Jacqueline in panic!

"How do I run this group? Where shall I aim it?" I asked.

Jacqueline gave me the perfect answers to get me started. I felt quite nervous about it but knew I could offer a positive mindset to help. I had gone through the journey myself - I definitely had a lot to offer. I had been on the other side of cancer, and this was a way of developing my new business, getting experience and exposure; the driving force to overcome public speaking. It would also allow me to develop short courses. An appearance on a local radio show allowed me to promote the wonderful work I was sharing. Little did I realise, as I had started at White House Cancer Support, that I was about to receive a message from the other side that would completely change how I would run these relaxation/meditation sessions in the future. My concern with public speaking was about to change.

What I didn't realise, was how this was about to play out within a couple of months ...

***

I truly believe in messages from the other side. I've experienced many of them. I have various stories from my own experiences of phenomenon. Most of them lovely, but also ones that have been quite concerning and frightening to me. I'm not saying this to get you concerned in any way or form, but these messages and phenomenon do exist. I've experienced being at places such as museums or stately homes where I've picked up some *'energy'* or frequency. I'm good at that - remember EHS! I get an idea of what has gone on there. It comes through as a gut instinct. Something which I have learned to follow more recently in life, and, as I have found out many times, it's usually true.

I'll give you a brief example. One visit I especially remember was at the 'Black Country Museum'. It's a local museum in Dudley quite near to us. I was around 17 at the time. I walked into one of the old houses, it was the kitchen part of the house. There were lots of pots and pans, black in colour, as were most of the things in that room, it was very dull. As I was standing there, I had this sudden thought appear in my mind, it said 'GET OUT!' It just seemed like a thought in my own mind. I initially disregarded it and continued looking at the room, but it came again. Starting to feel very uncomfortable, I urgently felt the need to leave the room and literally ... 'GET OUT' of there.

I said to the person I was with ... *"I really need to get out of here, I feel really uncomfortable."*

Once I'd left the building the feeling disappeared. After leaving the room, I was inquisitive to find out if I would experience the same feelings again if I went back in. So, I attempted to re-enter, but I just couldn't go back in. I couldn't even step over the door. How weird was that?

I have clairsalience abilities. Clairsalience is clear smelling. If you are tuned into this and aware of it, smells can often appear when a deceased family member is attempting to make connect with you. For example, smells associated with your deceased relative or friend. These could be things such as their perfume, or the smell of smoking that reminds you of them. Spirits and deceased can communicate with us in many ways if we become attuned to it, trusting what we are experiencing. My paternal grandmother communicates with me in this way. She has also moved objects and switched things on and off such as my washing machine. My washing machine ended up in the middle of the utility room right from under the worksurface at one point, and no, it wasn't switched on, nor had it done a load of washing - it was just there! It used to switch on and off playing a tune so that you knew it had finished. I often would hear it switch on, to which I would go and address it. This may sound ridiculous, but I used to stand in the room and say ... *'Hello nan, thank you for letting me know you are there. Hope you are ok. Everything is fine here. If it is you, please show me a sign.'* The washing machine would then instantly switch itself off! I would then respond with ... *'Thank you'* and leave the room. No, I haven't lost the plot talking to my washing machine - this genuinely happened and many times. Sadly, since my new washing machine has been fitted, it hasn't happened - but there is time yet. Nan connecting in doesn't happen a lot, but when she does, it is so powerful and brings me to tears. Usually, I find Nan communicates with me when I am experiencing a bad time in my life. It is as though my nan sends a message to reassure me; to let me know she's near and supporting me in the background. She especially did this before my diagnosis of cancer, sending me a hug of unconditional love - I felt the love being wrapped around me, it was very reassuring. Many psychic people I know have said she stands behind me and is with me, looking over me. I have had many things happen around our house. I could tell many stories; I just know it's my nan making that contact.

I was always very close to both my grandmothers and lucky enough to have them in my life for many years. Sadly, my dad's mom passed in October 1998 when I was 28. My other nan - my mom's mom - passed away in December 2016. She was 99 years old, about to reach her 100th birthday 5 months later. I was 46 at the time, we shared the same birthday date.

I distinctly remember the day my dad's mom passed. She had been unwell for quite a while - bedridden at home. Obviously, being bedridden causes the dreaded bed sores. She was suddenly taken ill and had to go into hospital. Sadly, it ended up being septicaemia and within a matter of days she passed. The day she passed; I was at home on my own just pottering about sorting housework etc. Suddenly, I had the urge to get on our electronic organ and play. Now this wasn't a usual thing for me, it wasn't my usual way to practise. I was in the middle of housework, but I just had this strong urge to stop and play music. Whilst learning electronic organ as a teenager, Nan used to keep asking me to play the song 'Eternally'[1] from a specific book. The words of the song go ... *'I'll be loving you eternally, with a love that's true, eternally'.* There were various songs in that book which she loved but especially liked this particular one. On the day of her passing, I suddenly realised that I had reached for this book which hadn't been off my music bookshelf for ages - years in fact. In an unconscious response, I opened the book and found myself playing 'Eternally'. I was also playing other songs from the book but, was especially drawn to this particular song. This had happened at a subconscious level - like I'd been guided to play this song with no control over it. Not long after stopping playing, the house telephone rang, it was my mom. She broke the news to me that Nan had passed.

"Are you sitting down?"

"Yes, I am. She's gone, hasn't she?" I responded.

At the moment Nan left this time - space - reality, I was playing those songs. Perfect timing! So, why did I get that strong urge to just stop what I was doing and play at that specific time, when I wouldn't usually do that? All I can put that down to is that my nan was making contact. I was serenading her during her passing. How amazing is that! I might be completely wrong here, but it seems way too coincidental to me for it not to be. Nothing is coincidental in life. This reassured me, helping me deal with her passing. A few weeks later, Karl had just left for work, I was still in bed. Aaron - who was around 9 months old - started to disturb in his cot. I was half asleep and suddenly heard ... sssshhhhh ... sssshhhhh ... coming from the baby monitor. I was tired and needed rest. Aaron settled down. As I thought about it later, once I'd woken up, I realised what I'd heard. I'm convinced it was my nan comforting Aaron so I could rest.

December 2016. It's here where things were about to play out how I least expected. The passing of my mom's mom, at 99, was a turning point for me. I was heartbroken when she passed but found I couldn't cry too deeply about it. After all, 99 years is an amazing age to reach! Her passing was more a celebration of her life - and what a long one she'd had at that! Nan had seen so much change over her life span; that is certainly something to be blessed with. Even recovering from bowel cancer 6 years before - we even went through cancer together! She had made the decision to not have an operation because of her age, but I convinced her to go ahead stating the truth ... *"Nan, if you don't have the op, you'll be dead by Christmas! You've got nothing to lose and everything to gain. You have had a good innings! If you die on the operating table, you won't have suffered, but if you survive the op, you could make a 100!"* Needless to say, she took my advice - changed her mind - had the op and survived.

My Uncle asked if there was anyone who would like to do a eulogy at her funeral. My instant reaction was *'Yes!'* I had an instant gut feeling flow through me to stand up and pay my respects to my nan. I don't even know where it came from. Normally, I'm a person who backs away from situations like that, especially public speaking or playing the piano in front of people - I just avoid it to be honest. I've always seen myself as a teacher rather than a performer. Back to the ... when I do put my mind to anything, I **can** do it, I know that deep down. But, through life, I seem to avoid those types of situations. What was fascinating, was the determination that came through me to do this for my nan. It felt so important, like there was another reason for it. That reason was about to make itself known to me.

I carefully planned my eulogy, including many happy memories. One important memory that needed to be included in my dedication was when Nan used to sing the song 'Que Sera Sera'[2] to me. While staying for sleep overs at my nan's, I remember her singing this song beautifully and so vividly, serenading me to sleep. She also used to sing 'Y Viva España'[3]. Especially singing it as she ventured off on her holidays abroad back in the 1970s. She loved her holidays to Spain back in the 70s, 80s and 90s. I even went on holiday with her and my auntie in 1987, flying for the first time at age 17. I loved it!

Careful planning of my dedicated words ended up being three pages long! The day of the funeral arrived. As I arrived at the church everyone kept asking if I was ok, and that if I didn't want to do the eulogy it was fine. Under the circumstances it was a hard thing to do.

The vicar said ... *"When it's your turn to stand up and speak Michelle, I'll look at you and nod my head. If you can nod back to say you are happy to do your eulogy, then I'll know you are going ahead. If not, that's ok, as people do feel they can't do these things on the day".*

I replied *"Thank you, but I'll be ok. I feel so determined. I want to do this for my nan."*

The time came for me to stand up and speak. I felt a feeling of inspiration, the strong urge to do it continued. I didn't know where this was coming from. I'd never felt so strongly about doing something! I wasn't even nervous, which is saying something for me! Especially as I was planning to sing 'Que Sera Sera' acapella and I'm not even a singer! While I was talking, I had this feeling come over me - I felt someone was guiding me, helping me. I felt it was my nan. After telling the story of 'Que Sera Sera', I invited the congregation to sing along with me. I just stood and sang. I remained calm throughout, my voice never faltered. I spoke powerfully and clear, with emotion and conviction. I could hear the vicar - who was to the right-hand side of me - singing with me, but I couldn't quite hear anyone in the congregation. It seemed like I was out there on my own. People later told me that they were singing along too. It really was all very bizarre, but wonderful, and certainly a true celebration of my dear nan's life.

So, what developed from that day? What changed in me? Since that day, I have to say I have completely changed. In the weeks and months that followed, I found I no longer got worked up or anxious about talking in front of people. I now speak clearly and confidently. I run my support groups and presenting myself doesn't bother me. That is something that I never thought I would, or could do. I also started doing 'Facebook lives' for a while for my business - that is definitely something I never thought I'd do - being live on the spot! You can't make a mistake - if you do, you must keep going. It did me the world of good.

So, from this point, things changed in quite a big way for me. As a holistic therapist now, I flow much better when I don't plan things. I speak from the heart, my gut instinct. I know I am guided in any moment. Having the experience of that day, at my nan's funeral, has aided and nourished this part of me - this part of communication. It has supported me in so many ways that I never believed possible. I do genuinely believe my nan was communicating with me, to do a eulogy, to stand up, to sing, just like my other nan connected sending reassurance from the other side to strengthen something within me. How amazing is that!

To this day, I still miss them both so much, but I know they are always near, keeping a look out for me.

A Way Will Be Found

We all have the ability to connect on different levels. Whether it be a reality level, or a spiritual level. Some people may disagree about connecting with spirit, but when we learn that everything is *'energy'*, we learn to process our understanding of the outside world differently, bringing it into our inner world - a world of deep connection. We are all connected. There are always plenty of signs out there, showing us and guiding us. We just have to learn to look out for them, tune into them, look and learn from our gut instinct, and use our intuition for these messages - which can be shown to us in many ways. Think of the robin that appears outside your kitchen window to say hello. How many people trust that a dear one is near when they see a robin close by? It's the same type of thing. Learning to have an awareness of that possibility triggers a more 'tuned in' perception - then you start to find coincidences happening. Of course, you'll question them, but then you'll start to see that there are no such things as coincidences.

What did I learn from that December day back in 2016? How can we look at this from a place of realignment? Why do we continue to create fears?

'Fear' always seems to pop its ugly head up just when you don't want it to doesn't it? We are here understanding FEAR again! There is nothing to fear! Only our thoughts about any situation can create fear within us. Where does fear come from? We are only born with two fears - the fear of loud noises and the fear of falling - so why do we create such fears? Understanding thoughts associated with our experiences allows us to foster a different perspective, thus allowing us to change our responses as fears creep in. We can take a step back, change the thoughts in our mind's eye before that fear develops into something more.

I love Eckhart Tolle's quote, which states the obvious regarding our thoughts. Until you stop and think about your thoughts, you don't even realise what you are doing ...

'What a liberation to realise that the "voice in my head" is not who I am.
Who am I then? The one who sees that.'[4]

Everything starts with a thought. Thoughts create things. A thought creates a feeling or emotion within us. From that feeling or emotion we take action. From that action, we experience the outcome or reality of the original thought. Every thought you think works like this. Having the realisation that thought is the exact starting point at which we create our reality, means we can start to change it. It's only our thoughts about anything that triggers responses. Those responses come from our past experiences. This is where our subconscious mind thinks it's protecting us, wanting to do the right thing for us, because that is all it knows. Our subconscious can only work with its original training, using the same old responses, which it has already practised. But if the subconscious doesn't understand time, is it really holding onto the past? Is it really connected to it? The subconscious only works with NOW, it doesn't apply logic. It lives in the part of the brain that is opposite to logic, the monkey brain. Which is why we create stories that bring fear for ourselves.

So ... are we connected to our past? Most people will say 'yes'. But are we really? How are we connected to those past experiences? It's a difficult question for people to answer. We are indeed, only connected to our past by the 'thoughts' we hold around it - our memories. The thought brings past experiences into the NOW - we know that's all the subconscious has ... NOW! When we understand what's going on, we can start to change those responses, especially ones around fear.

Those messages from the other side became one of the best realisations for me, allowing me to release *'fear'*. Each moment was a new NOW and I had control over it. It's only when we let go of the past, that we can move from FEAR to FREEDOM!

References:

1. Parsons, G., & Turner, J. (1953). *Eternally*. [Recorded by] Young, J.

2 Livingston, J., & Evans, R. (1955). *Que Sera Sera*. [Recorded by] Day, D.

3 Caerts, L., & Rozenstraten, L. (1971). *Y Viva España*. [Recorded by] Bervoets, C.

4 Tolle, E. (2005). *A New Earth: Awakening to Your Life's Purpose*. Penguin Books.

Michelle Townsend

Chapter 20

Becoming Who I Am

'If there's something you want to master but it makes you nervous, do it as much as you can! The only way to learn is to do it! ... Follow your heart.'

~ Michelle Townsend

Who was I developing into? What transformations had happened to me in a short amount of time? I felt a different person if I'm being completely honest. Thinking back to what I had learnt and continued to learn was phenomenal - there was so much! I was also finding myself in different situations, making choices that I never would have made.

A friend, Ian, helped get me started building my website *'harmonylifebalance.co.uk'*[1] - also creating my logo of *'three white and black butterflies'*, symbolising body-mind-spirit connection, for which I am very grateful. The number 3 has always been relevant in my life - thus represented in my logo. *'White butterflies'* symbolise spiritual transformation, *'black butterflies'* renewal, change and hope in the face of adversity. I continued to learn how to add information to my website. Voluntary work was becoming important to me, as well as building my new business of 'Harmony Life Balance'[1]

Hypnotherapy. This led me to train in First Degree Reiki. I also started working for 'Salus Fatigue Foundation'[2], running courses about the mind-body connection and understanding the mind - helping people with chronic fatigue. I kept developing - connecting into the real me. I was getting what I focused on! Like attracts Like! Vibrating at the same frequency! Attracting where I was focused. Everything was flowing and falling into place, but there were still aspects of my life that needed changing, adjusting.

2017 arrived. In the years from 2010 through to 2017 I'd had the approach ... *'I'm going to live my life to its fullest.'* I'd gone through all this trauma - so why not? This included eating what I enjoyed and wanted, eating out a lot, holidays and socialising. I also started to enjoy alcohol more. Alcohol had never really floated my boat! I'd never had any interest in it in my younger years, couldn't see the point. Then, red wine suddenly became a very nice drink to complement a meal out. Even our boys commented ... *'Don't you think you are drinking too much mom?'* They had never seen me drink, so to them, a couple of glasses made me look an alcoholic! From all these choices, I piled the weight on. By Christmas 2016, I was the heaviest I had ever been in my whole life. I had reached over 13 and a half stone - heavier than my full-term pregnancies! Life was good, but I noticed aches in my hips, I didn't feel comfortable and I felt inflammation in my body.

April 2017 saw me addressing what I ate. 'Salus' had highlighted how important food was in healing the body. I had already had a cortisol injection into my right hip, to help with the pain - I couldn't lie on my hips, they were keeping me awake. Was it the after-effects of chemotherapy catching up with me? By the September, I was advised to go gluten, dairy and egg free - also being told to leave out soya, sugar and yeast, as I had also been suffering with symptoms of candida, a common ailment from chemotherapy treatment. It was time to make changes. Within two weeks of removing these foods out of my diet, I had lost 2 stone. The weight just dropped off me … literally! Ever attempted taking all those foods out in one foul swoop? It's hard! The worst one being sugar. They put sugar in pretty much everything! I was frustrated by food. What could I eat? Eating out was difficult. Trips to the supermarket were becoming a nightmare, we were having to check what everything contained. I wanted to be healthy, protecting my body by eating healthily. Eventually, Karl and I knew what I could eat and it became less of an issue. It was back to the raw basics - vegetables and food in its natural state. By the time we visited New York in February 2018, I was down to 8 stone 9lbs. I'd gone from size 14 to size 8/10. I felt amazing! The pain and inflammation had left my body, my hips were no longer an issue, nor was the candida which had been part of the inflammation problem since cancer. I felt a new lease of life! I felt I had a new body yet again. Thy food is thy medicine!

Then, in **March 2017**, I went to a talk by Dr David Hamilton, writer of the book 'How Your Mind Can Heal Your Body'[3]. More things were being shown to me. Dr David Hamilton's book was reassurance of everything I had put in place for my healing regarding my mind work - yet I hadn't been aware of his books before now. He had also written a book called 'It's The Thought That Counts'[4]. Obviously, I was drawn in straight away. He was on my wavelength, it all made perfect sense.

It was around this time, that I became more aware of my hearing deteriorating, but only in my right ear. I had always had tinnitus since a teenager from listening to loud music in headphones, but it seemed to be getting worse. When lying in bed on my left side, I couldn't hear much through my right ear, it was very limited. I had issues making out consonants, which start and end words. This makes it difficult to understand what people are saying, especially in social places where there are lots of people talking. I was finding I was agreeing to what people were saying, but hadn't a clue what they had said! This was also happening during Covid times when people wore masks. I suddenly realised how much I lip read! The type of chemotherapy treatment I received could cause hearing loss, usually in one ear - weird I know! After a hearing test, I was told I qualified for a hearing aid in my right ear only. At first, I was given a hearing aid that was moulded to my ear. It felt old-fashioned, not the very small 'receiver in ear canal' (RIC) that pushed right into my ear, where it looked hidden. The audiologist said the RIC hearing aid wouldn't work for my type of hearing loss. This new hearing aid looked obvious, with a big tube running behind my ear. I found I wasn't wearing it much. After returning for my check-ups, I was later told a RIC hearing aid would work for me, and she couldn't understand why I hadn't been given one in the first place. *'Great!'* I thought ... *'I've only had this old fashioned looking one for 3 years - I've hardly wore it.'* A new RIC hearing aid was set up for me and I have never looked back since. It's amazing! Words are much clearer now. The amazing thing is, is my new hearing-aid has Bluetooth ... yes - Bluetooth! It connects to my phone - I can take phone calls through it - listen to music through it - watch YouTube etc. I wear it in my right ear all day - every day. That would not have been a possibility back in the days of EHS. It would have freaked me out completely. Proof of powerful change - I did it!

April 2018 saw the arrival of my new car. I had always wanted an Abarth 595 Convertible. I'd enjoyed my little Fiat 500C, so changed it for a red Abarth. It was great! The thing was, both these cars had Bluetooth. I was now owning cars with Bluetooth fitted and using the connections. WOW! Initially, when I had new cars slight EHS symptoms appeared, it seemed I had to address the EHS. I would instantly work with my *'OK technique',* acknowledge it, then change the thought process around the responses. EHS would then disappear! *'Fear'* no longer resided here. It was like it would appear to remind me how far I'd come. Well, that's how I perceived it. But was my response because of the new way I was dealing with it, the way I now perceived the EHS? Afterall, 'it's the thought that counts.' Thought creates the responses - placebo effect! It's never been a problem from then on, those responses haven't happened with cars we have had ever since. Again, probably because I addressed it straight away and didn't feed it. I just accepted and let go, believing *'it's ok'*.

March 2020. Covid struck! Pupils and clients were no longer allowed in my home. My only option was to move all work online. This also proved an extremely big turning point for me. 'Zoom' appeared - so I set in place the facility to *'zoom-in'* to teach online. It was all very daunting at first, not knowing how it was all going to work, would I lose clients? Would I be able to teach online all the time? Initially, EHS never really crossed my mind, I don't think about it much nowadays, but after a few weeks of teaching online I did have a few slight responses - just like I'd had when changing my cars. It appeared to say hello in my arms and chest area. Once again, I addressed the responses with *'OK technique'* - it then faded into nothingness yet again. Work was less busy during covid and like many people during that time I lost a lot of my earnings, but we got through it. I was just so glad that I had my online options to continue at least a little. I still teach online lessons to this day; it changed my way of teaching.

As May appeared, my 50th wasn't how I'd planned it. My 3-week cruise to the North Cape had been cancelled - as with all cruises, but we had a fabulous 'online Zoom Party', of which Karl did an amazing job of organising. I mean ... 'online!' This would never have been possible with EHS! Karl prepared music quizzes such as, 'name that tune', 'name the advert', plus many more. Thank heavens for 'online!' We later celebrated my 50th birthday in November 2021-18 months later - at our local Indian restaurant. It was fabulous! I declared that I hadn't reached 50 until I'd had my face-to-face 50th party.

As we travelled through the lockdowns, a breast cancer scare in July 2020 threw me into turmoil. I found indents on the side of my right breast. My responses weren't what I would have expected. After all I had gone through and learnt about the mind-body-connection, I thought I would have dealt with it in a much more positive way. Instead, I went into panic mode, worrying, thinking the worst. I didn't really want a mammogram because they are so invasive. I couldn't wait - so I paid private to have breast thermography from 'Medical Thermography.'[5] It is a compression-free - non-invasive - radiation-free - pain-free - no-contact procedure. It is infrared technology, which can detect abnormal vascular activity in breast tissue. Thankfully, further tests showed all was clear, but the shock and stress upset my system. It took me a while to bring back balance. I was disappointed in myself that I didn't deal with it the way I thought I should have; like in 2010 with Hodgkin's Lymphoma and of course EHS. Needless to say, apart from this scare, we had a good summer that year, blessed with wonderful weather. It made the lockdowns more manageable.

Aaron had moved back home. Aaron was in his final year at 'Royal Welsh College of Music' in Cardiff studying percussion. Ethan in his last year of college, before leaving for university. Both boys had been accepted into 'Royal College of Music' (RCM) in London - Aaron a Masters in percussion, Ethan a 4-year Degree in saxophone. We were gutted things ended so abruptly for them before leaving for London. As the lockdowns progressed further, the house had to be adjusted for all 4 of us. Aaron completing his final performance in Ethan's bedroom on a 5-octave marimba via Zoom - Karl was teaching online - I was teaching online - we needed more powerful Wi-Fi in the house! We already had two routers, with one in my music room, which I was using. So, we invested in three boosters - we had to, we were all online! Again, a small thought came into the back of my mind about EHS, but this time, I had no problems at all with the frequencies. I was so proud of myself! Eventually, in September, both Aaron and Ethan ventured off to start their next educational steps in London at RCM. We were so proud of them both.

A Way Will Be Found

Over the years, my various responses regarding EHS, and these little 'relapses' made me think further. Obviously, I wasn't too happy about them, but after stopping to think for a while…. this was GREAT! *Let's look at this in a different perspective. Relapses are good for you, giving you a kick up the back side, keeping you on your toes! It's also, a reminder of how far you've come!'* A relapse allowed me to see how far I'd moved forward. Without it, I couldn't see the contrast of positive change gained. *'If you can do it once, you can do it again'* - instilling in me to keep going - looking at what I've achieved so far - strengthening rather than knocking me down. It was, in fact, more than GREAT! It was the preparation taking place - EHS relapses had prepared me for my cancer journey. This was the proof I needed regarding the contents of my book! The relapses drove me to believe more and more about everything I had researched - 'law of attraction' - 'creating our own reality', and having the power to create change - it was becoming my TRUTH my UNDERSTANDING. Obviously, I'd had many doubts about it, who wouldn't? These experiences answered my questions fully; reaffirming that I was, indeed, on the right track. These relapses allowed me to strengthen my beliefs and responses around the effects of EHS every time they reappeared in some way, no matter how small. It was *'practise…practise…practise!'*

Over the years, there were times where I did no writing at all, working through that low *'energy'* space, especially cancer. I needed proof. Time to prove that what I was about to write was genuine and worked! I understand now that my experiences were all meant to be, even right up to now. I played with the mind work - played with the responses, feelings and emotions. I accepted all experiences as positive situations that were necessary for the completion of this book. I allowed my body to do what it had to do. The symptoms came and went many times, but my observation of them was critical and changed each time. Initially, this could have made things worse for me because of my beliefs about creating reality. Was I sending out the frequency to keep experiencing the symptoms because I was aware of them? They were, after all, continuously changing - I had released the 'fear'.

Having experienced complete cure from this debilitating dis-ease of EHS was what kept me focused. The stress and worry that came with the first experience of EHS was no longer there. My mind was responding differently. I now looked at relapses in a positive manner and utilised the experience to its fullest. Now was my chance to get my thoughts and responses just right, to help others. These relapses highlighted ...

- You are an electromagnetic being.
- Everything in the universe is electromagnetic vibrating at its own very special frequency.
- Matter is created through the frequency at which atoms vibrate together.
- Thought creates matter.
- Looking for something that exists, usually creates that something in your experience - your perception.
- The <u>expectation</u> of that something happening, sends out the frequency, most likely creating this in your experience.
- You <u>create your own reality</u> (1963)[6].

I came to understand, that knowing these very crucial important points helped to turn things around. Not only with EHS, but with anything. This is how the universe responds to thought. I then went on to realise ...

- A new reality can exist. Trust it.

- Accept your experience - not judge it as a bad experience - just accept, knowing a change can come forth. (Use me as an example if you wish - the lady who cured EHS by focusing on a new reality).

- Your current situation is the residue of past thoughts relating to any dis-ease you experience. You **do** have a choice to change your thoughts.

- Visualize how you want your life experience to be. Sometimes, it helps to not think about the situation at hand and just focus on nature, beautiful things that make you smile and relax. Keep your focus simple. Being grateful for what you already have in your life is helpful. Practise *'gratitude'*. By focusing on something that already exists removes the frequency of what you don't have, to what you do have. Proving you can manifest in your experience. That's the same with anything in life. We all create what's around us by our thoughts, choices and decisions.

- Create the feeling of having what you want now. Imagine what it is you are wanting happening now, as if it has already happened in your life experience. Your subconscious mind does not distinguish between real or imaginary. Your bodily functions react the same either way. Your subconscious mind does not associate with time. It believes what you are seeing or thinking to be happening right NOW!

- Tell your new story how you want it to be, as though it has already happened. This can be extremely hard.

Your body will create the experience about what you talk about the most. If you find the subject matter uncomfortable, just don't mention it for quite a while - don't broach the subject - just like I made the decision to stop talking about my symptoms. When people ask, just say ... 'it's sorted now!' You're not lying, because you have sorted it. You have chosen to change your thoughts about it - there lies a big change in itself.

- The frequency emanating from your body is reflecting out into the universe attracting like frequencies back to you that match perfectly. So, the thoughts you should be sending out are how you want things to be right now, in this present moment. Trust from an understanding of quantum mechanics, that thought frequency precedes matter. Trust in this. Watch the changes.

- What have you got to lose? No doubt you have felt or are feeling hopeless about this situation. So, you therefore have nothing to lose but everything to gain anyway! Use the feeling of hopelessness to let go of the situation. This is *'acceptance'*. It is most likely you will see an improvement straight away because you have let go of the resistance. Surrender to it. Completely.

When I started looking back, the process of breaking these realisations down, and honouring them, took me to another level of understanding. It developed me further. Bringing forward that reassurance to continue this path of mind power. I realised how important it was in *'becoming who I am'*. When the occasional symptoms of EHS crept back in, it was nothing major, it just made itself aware - new cars, zoom, etc... but in my mind, I knew and trusted I had sorted it! My belief had changed, I was now running a new updated 'app'!

References:

1. Townsend, M. (2016) *Harmony Life Balance.*
   https://www.harmonylifebalance.co.uk

2. *Salus Fatigue Foundation.* https://www.salus.org.uk

3. Hamilton, D. (2008). *How Your Mind Can Heal Your Body.*
   Hay House.

4. Hamilton, D. (Original text 2005). (2008). *It's the Thought
   That Counts.* Hay House.

5. *Medical Thermography.* https://medscans.co.uk

6. Roberts, J. (Original text 1963). *The Early Sessions. Book 1.
   The Seth Material.*

Michelle Townsend

Chapter 21

Learning to Flow

'You know you've let go of the past when the anniversary of the date passes you by and you don't even realise it.'

~ Michelle Townsend

How was I learning to flow? Allowing myself to live my life? No longer holding onto the past? I was talking with a friend during the writing of this book, when it came up in conversation about the day I was diagnosed with cancer. Suddenly, I realised that the date of its anniversary had passed by only 6 days before. The previous week had gone by without me even realising! Initially, I was aware of the anniversary the first few years after 26th January 2010, but for quite a few years now, it passes without any realisation. Even looking in my diary doesn't register it for me, it's not on my wavelength.

I stopped to think about this more as the conversation went on.

I said to my friend ... *"I really have let that go haven't I? I no longer hold onto the memory of that life changing day."*

I felt quite proud of myself in that moment of realisation. It's so important to live in the NOW! What's passed is past, we can't change it, we can only learn from it. Using the adversity to guide us forward with wisdom. Living in memories and anniversaries of these types of dates only holds it there, keeping us connected to the memories. Move on, it's just a space in time. That was then, this is NOW!

The realisation highlighted the importance of honouring the memory when becoming aware of such dates. To be proud of what I went through and got through, then let it go. Savour NOW, living NOW!

I asked myself ... *'What anniversaries do I hold onto? How do I think about them? Are they negative or positive? What do I gain from it?'* This awareness changed the way I saw the past.

Coming to an understanding that we are dying from the day we are born, we can see life through a different lens. I'm not being negative here, just highlighting a fact. It's true! Learn to savour each and every special moment - good and bad. We move through life thinking it all just happens the way it does and have no say in the matter - but we are the directors of our story - we can direct it - do direct it - we do have choices. Unfortunately, people are not necessarily aware of these choices or think about it in this way.

Cancer journeys can trigger us to realise the most important things in life. To choose what we truly want, savouring who we are at any point in our lives, in any *'now'* moment. This refocuses us on what we truly want from our lives. Do we need all the materialistic things? Or are our experiences and memories more important to us?

Just like my cancer journey triggered a new direction in me - a new career; there are people out there, when put in life changing situations, discard the old rat race, replanting themselves in a place they want to be. Why did they not do that from the beginning? Why did they not look at life with themselves as the director before? Choosing what they truly want in the first place? Everything happens for a reason. It's usually where we are focused. Direct it!

Yes, we need certain materialistic things in our life to make our life comfortable, but there's a lot we don't need. Sometimes simplicity is so much better. Do we need keepsakes? I always used to keep things for best, for a special day. *'I won't use it; I'll keep it for best,'* I would say. Every day is special, every day is our best day. One day that special best day will be our last. Live each day as though it's your last!

When we learn to let go of physical objects, we open ourselves up to *'freedom'.* We no longer live in *'fear'* of losing those physical things. With no *'fear'* there's *'freedom'*.

In **May 2021**, the realisations continued to flow. 12 months on from my 50th birthday, I treated myself to an Apple iWatch without even thinking about the Bluetooth connections and what the iWatch does. Within the first two weeks of wearing it, I had unusual pains in my arm, it was aching. So, once again, I addressed the EHS - spoke to it - had a chat with it - just like I had done with all that had affected me before. Again, *'fear'* no longer resided here. Within 24 hours of addressing the EHS, the symptoms vanished. I have been wearing my iWatch everyday ever since, with no issues. This reaffirmed to me that I was running that new program in my subconscious mind, I trusted the addressing of EHS wholeheartedly. I believed the process, so it became my reality. It was great I could use it. The iWatch encouraged Karl and I to take up running. Using the 'Activity' function, we decided to start the 'Couch to 5K'. July appeared, and whilst away in North Wales, we started the programme. Working with the 'app', we flowed through each week's target goal, developing us further. By December 2021, I was running 5K in just under 33 minutes. I couldn't believe it! Originally, I couldn't even run across a road without my knees hurting, let alone consider 5K ... but I did it! I was always a hopeless runner at school - nearly keeling over when running round the school playing fields. I was now using every experience as an opportunity for growth. Although running has stopped and started since then, I know I can do it. Achieving things I believed I couldn't, encourages me on to other new experiences - building confidence to give it a go, no matter what the outcome. What's important here, was the fun in the experience, not the Apple iWatch, or the 'app' - it was spending time with Karl and friends running, 'enjoying the moment' - that was my top priority now.

It's these 'enjoying the moment' times that were important during Covid times. With all of us being at home, our beautiful dog Tess, had all the love she could ask for around her. She got used to us being home all the time. In hindsight, this was all meant to be. October 2021 brought shock that we weren't expecting at all. A tumour on Tess's spleen, which we never knew about ruptured. She had only just gone 8. Sadly, it was her time to go. The loss was to break our hearts. She had reinforced to me, the understanding of 'energetic connection'. Tess, who I called my 'little sidekick', helped me with clients who had a fear of dogs. She healed so many people in the time she was with us. Tess was very 'tuned in' to people's *energy* - either gently approaching, or keeping away if she knew they were fearful. Pupils' parents who had a fear of dogs fell in love with her, overcoming their fears, going on to own dogs of their own. Tess helped hypnotherapy clients overcome their fears, she worked with me in a powerful way. So many young children grew to love her when they visited. Sadly, she left us too soon. Tess was a true healer.

After attending the 'International Hypnotherapy Association's Conference' a few days before Tess's passing, I signed up for the 'Hypno-Oncology Practitioner Course'[1] with Garry Coles - and by February 2022, I qualified as a Hypno-Oncology Practitioner. This allowed me to further develop my hypnotherapy skills, working specifically with cancer patients - using hypnotherapy to help them on their cancer journey, supporting their psychological well-being. Mindset is so important - the mind-body connection helps with the healing process. I had first-hand experience of being on the other side of cancer. Hypnotherapy had been the turning point for me back in 2010, and this course was helping me offer so much more. My hypnotherapy business was now developing well.

A Way Will Be Found

We are here for the ride of our life no matter what it may be - it's not about completing anything. When we realise that we never stop learning, we can take on a different approach to life. Many of us think, that when we have completed something, we come to a point where we think we are done. I call it the *'completion'* feeling. I've had this feeling many times, especially as a young adult. When I experience it now, I find I laugh at myself, because I now know I'll never stop learning. It took me a long time to realise this believe it or not. I know that may sound like complete balderdash! It's a common feeling within many humans. What's important to remember is...WE are never done! WE are always evolving! Right up until we decide to leave this current time-space-reality. Taking the approach of always moving forward ... that we will never be complete ... opens many doors for us. This changes our perspective to just aim and continue to learn. I think schooling gives this outlook of learning. When you leave school, you're done! 'Been there got the t-shirt' feeling - done all the learning! Even though we've finished school, our knowledge of learning doesn't stop. It is never too late to learn anything. It's never too late to start again. Age is irrelevant! We are all big kids at heart. We can go on to do anything and achieve whatever we feel inspired to do. Louise Hay didn't establish Hay House[2] Publishing firm until she was 58!

Then there's the ... why do we so often go through life not appreciating what we've already achieved? We just get on the tread mill and keep going - not necessarily thinking anything is a real achievement - only focusing on the big things as a success. Life itself is a journey and an achievement! You are here creating your life, creating the learning. Whether there are good times, bad or sad times, we are here to enjoy and learn from each step of the journey of life.

Remembering to honour each of the little things as big achievements ... because they are achievements ... is important. It's the little things that all add up - building on the experience. Where we initially start, isn't where we eventually end up. I didn't know EHS would be a blessing in disguise, preparing my mind for cancer, creating the understanding of mind - I didn't know how my cancer journey would pan out, but I survived - I didn't know how I was going to run my relaxation group to help support cancer patients initially; but over time, it has developed into something I am very proud of with more and more people attending and loving it! Living their best life possible. I'm so proud of the people who attend my group, using their adversity to create powerful change - 5k wasn't possible but became possible. No matter what your achievements be grateful for them all. When we come from a place of *'gratitude'* in life, everything is special and an achievement - even getting out of bed that day! Honour that! That's an experience to be grateful for.

It's important to honour any adversity as guidance and wisdom. Rather than getting drawn into negativity for too long, change it. Honour those fears, for we create them. *'Fear'* can be transformational! Acknowledge the situation. Ask what the situation is teaching you and then move on. You'll make choices and decisions that you would never have considered before if it hadn't have happened...and that's a good thing!! That's the journey of *'becoming who you are!'* ... **'A way will be found!'**

So, stop and take a moment...because you are AMAZING!! Where can you take the next step of your journey? What turns you on? What are you drawn to?

Time to grab your journal and a pen. Here's a few questions you can ask yourself about becoming who you are - continuing that 'self-development'. Write down your answers - be completely honest with yourself. It may change your life!

- What are my achievements that I am proud of?
- What did I gain from those achievements?
- What new situations or experiences have arisen from those achievements?
- Where have these achievements inspired me to look?
- Have I followed that inspiration?
- Is that inspiration something I could investigate?
- What am I really interested in?
- Where do I feel my interests are being drawn to?
- Could I follow what I'm drawn to, to create a better life?
- What am I fearful of?
- What negative situations in my life ended up being a blessing in disguise?

How often do we ask ourselves these types of questions? We don't! Well ... some might, but not on a regular basis. **WE** should be asking these questions more often if we want to direct our life. We are not handed our life to just live it - **WE** direct it! Every single bit of it! If we can create change from our thoughts, asking these types of simple questions could allow us to make decisions that could be life changing - thus allow us to follow our heart, our intuition, our inner guidance, that *'inner child'*. Then you are truly *'becoming who you are'.* Life is a big adventure - go out and explore.

'When we deal with the energetic - and thoughts
are energetic, the physical responds.'

~ Michelle Townsend

References:

1. Coles, G. *Hypno-Oncology.* https://hypno-oncology.com
2. Hay, L. (Founded 1984, Carlsbad, California). *Hay House Publishers.* https://www.hayhouse.com

Chapter 22

A Way Will Be Found

'Even if you doubt ... even if you don't think you can do it!!
JUST DO IT!
No one initially knows how to do anything; we all have to learn
each and every step of the way. If we can adopt that JUST DO IT
mindset through life, then anything is possible!
... A Way Will Be Found!'

~ Michelle Townsend

Now, as a Hypnotherapist, the more I work with the mind the more it amazes me! I've experienced seeing fabulous changes in clients in sessions that just blow your mind away! Seeing these responses and changes in sessions, for me, is the reassurance that the mind certainly can create powerful change. Sometimes, in the very simplest of ways.

Nothing inspires me more than the feeling of helping someone. Maybe that's why my life's journey panned out the way it has. I also feel humbled when thinking how many music pupils I have helped over the years. Teaching them something they will always be able to tap into - 'music' - what a wonderful gift to have. I gave them that! WOW! Music at their fingertips. Look at what music creates for many people around the world. It is a universal language. Put musicians from different nationalities together to play the same piece of music and they all coordinate together creating a harmonious sound, even though they don't speak a word of each other's language! It creates 'communication.' There are always ways to connect.

Everything happens in divine timing. Things fall into place when the time is right for us. No one knows what tomorrow will bring. I have had a wonderful 14 years since my diagnosis of Hodgkin's Lymphoma - I don't know how many years I have left, no one does - wellness or illness is irrelevant! But what I am sure of - by keeping a positive mindset, is what has given me all these years post cancer - post chemotherapy treatment. It has highlighted to me to live each day the best way you can. Even days where you feel like locking yourself away and feel awful - even those days are special! They give us perspective and new direction. If we haven't got the contrast, we have nothing to compare to. Honour it fully.

Yes, I stress - yes, I worry - I proved that recently with a breast cancer scare - I am only human. Even this book has taken me further on my healing journey reminding me of how far I've come, facing fears I never thought existed!

It's in the 'challenging changes', those 'breaking points', those struggles of daily life, where we make our 'best decisions'. It's the 'practise … practise … practise', in finding our true strength - connecting with our 'trust … faith … belief', our 'inner child'. It's in those struggles we search for resources to help us in, 'becoming who we are' and 'learning to flow'. Life is unpredictable. It is what it is! Live each day as if it's the most important one. You never know what it might become when you do so. Just remember 'it's OK'.

The little moments of life are often the big moments - remember to savour them, don't miss them. My family get fed up with me taking so many photos - I drive them mad! Especially whilst out on a walk keep stopping to snapshot the beauty. But where do my family come when they want a photo of a memory or celebration? Me! I've got a photo for everything! Create those special images within your mind.

When we practise *'acceptance'* for our actions and responses, we learn so much more about ourselves. We all make mistakes, we are, after all, only following our natural *'human needs'* at any point in our life. But are those mistakes really mistakes? Ask yourself ... *'What did it teach me? Did it strengthen me in some way? What did I gain from the knowledge of that experience?'* No one deliberately goes out to hurt anyone - well that's the case for most. We do what feels right in any moment for ourselves, even helping others. We are filling that *'human need'* at any point in time. It is teaching us a lesson, to develop our soul expression, taking us to those *'times for a change'*. When we see it from that new perspective, it highlights that we come from a place of love - there is only love - there can only be that. We are all doing our best - flying by the seat of our pants everyday anyway!

So, when anyone does anything to you that feels uncomfortable, step back and ask yourself ... *'What are they attempting to fill in their life? What **'human need'** are they fulfilling? What is missing for them right now?'* Because usually, it's what's missing from their life that creates the action or response they gave. We all respond the best way we can from our own perspective, feelings and beliefs. Your choices are right for you - living in the NOW!

Learning to connect into the **'energy'** of believing in yourself - connecting with your aspirations - following your dreams - that's where the real **'you'**, your *'inner child'* will flow forward! Believe you really can do it! Ask questions of yourself - find out what you love. You've got to love what you do! When you love doing something, it will flow naturally, you won't need to struggle through it. Find out what turns you on and follow the feeling.

Life isn't always great, and sometimes we must work at it. Remember to *'use the adversity to create the change'* you want. Follow your heart - your gut instinct - you'll get better and better. You've got to believe in *'you'* because that's all you have ... *'YOU!'* Connect with that *'trust ... faith ... belief'* and *'A way will be found'*, moving yourself *'from fear to freedom'*.

Everything is *'energy!'* When we see it from this perspective, it all makes perfect sense. We can make things as difficult, or as easy as we like. Which *'energy'* do we choose? Are we choosing *'fear?'* ... or are we choosing *'freedom?'* It's simple - it's your choice - there's nothing more to it! When 'it's' simple *'a way will be found!'*

Epilogue

Aaron - now in his mid-twenties - lives north of London, doing what he enjoys - building his career in music. After graduating with Honours for his Master's from the 'Royal College of Music', Aaron gained a scholarship with 'Southbank Sinfonia' - spending a year with them based in Westminster, London. Aaron has developed into an astounding percussionist and never ceases to amaze us, turning up to gigs and sight-reading!

Ethan - now graduated from 'Royal College of Music' with a First Class Honours for his double degree in classical and jazz saxophone - is continuing and developing his interest in jazz at Masters level at the 'Royal Academy of Music'. Ethan's desire to compose his own music and progress as a jazz saxophonist shines through. His tonality and sound just flow harmoniously in his improvised jazz passages. A phenomenal player!

Aaron and Ethan both continue enjoying London and the opportunities it has given them. Karl and I are extremely proud of them. We continue to enjoy visiting them, attending many concerts whenever we can.

Lin Porter - my dear friend who gave me so much support all those years ago - sadly passed away suddenly and unexpectedly in September 2023, as I was finalising this book. It seems more relevant now than ever to dedicate *'From Fear to Freedom'* to Lin. She will always remain in my heart and my thoughts. I will always be thankful for her wonderful support, kind-heartedness and patience. Thank you.

Mike England remains a wonderful dear friend. Although our weekly meet-ups over the last few years haven't been as regular as we'd have wished, when we do meet, it is like we've never been apart - a true, deep friendship, that I honour and am truly grateful for. Mike, I owe my life to you. Thank you.

Julie my best friend from school remains a wonderful friend. We meet on a regular basis, especially loving our shopping trips! It was during one of our shopping trips that the title *'From Fear to Freedom'* was born. Julie continues to flourish in her own life and career, where she received the promotion she so wanted very recently. I'm so proud of you. Thank you for being 'you'. Keep being 'you'!

Both sets of parents are still with us, and although various ailments have slowed them down in recent years, they keep going. Karl, Aaron, Ethan and I feel extremely blessed to have them in our lives, and we continue to make special memories.

Now, making extra-special time to enjoy our holidays in Wales and on our cruises, Karl and I make the most of what we have, savouring all aspects of our lives.

Acknowledgements

My first thanks go to the three most important men in my life - my sons, Aaron and Ethan, and my husband Karl.

Aaron and Ethan - you have kept me focused by your love of music. The excitement I experience when I hear of your successes and your love for music has kept me going. I am so proud of the wonderful young men you have become. Keep doing what you love and enjoy!

Karl - I thank you for putting up with me! I cannot thank you enough for tolerating those rough times, for being patient when others would have left. You give me strength when I lose my focus, kicking me back into gear, reminding me to practise what I preach!

My family - I will always be indebted for all the love and support you have given me in those challenging times of need. I thank you for always being there by my side and your continued support to this day. Without you all, my life would have been very different.

Gratitude to my wonderful friends Julie and Claire for your tips on punctuation, grammar and proof-reading along this amazing journey. Your advice has been invaluable. Our friendships stand the true test of time. I feel blessed.

Special thanks go to Lynn Partridge - my amazing editor and proof-reader. Without you, this book would not be what it is today. Thank you for all the hours you have dedicated to this project, your patience and support - you kept me going when it all felt too much. I am eternally grateful. Thank you for being a wonderful friend.

I am very grateful to have had two amazing hypnotherapists in my life. Not only did Mike England play an important part in changing my life for the better, back in 2007, but he also helped support me through my training with Jacqueline Panchaud. I am forever indebted to you both for your amazing guidance along my journey. Thank you, you've been amazing!

To all the doctors and nurses on Georgina Unit at Russells Hall Hospital back in 2010, and the support that followed. I thank you so much.

My 'White House' family - you remind me of the strength I had back then. You are all truly amazing! Keep living your best lives! Thank you for being you and listening when I have voiced ideas regarding this book. It is, after all, about a cancer journey. I have appreciated and taken on board your feedback and continued support to make this happen.

Thanks and gratitude go to Ian Whitmore, for designing my butterfly logo back in 2016 and bringing my website to life. I still love the *'three white and black butterflies'* logo that you created from my idea, which was scribbled down in my own little artistic way back then! I continue to add content and update information on my website myself - it's been great to learn! Special thanks go to Darren Perks for keeping my website *'Harmony Life Balance'* updated - which I appreciate very much. Thanks also go to Emily Jones for working very swiftly when I needed my Mailing List set up for my Newsletter back in October 2022. Thank you all so much.

Special thanks go to Sharon Eddowes and David Jones regarding my book cover design. Your feedback has been invaluable. Thank you so much for listening and making me look at graphic design from a new perspective.

'White Magic Studios' - my self-publishing company. Thank you for your patience getting my book cover and typescript to what it is today. When alterations were needed, we manipulated and worked together. We got there!

Thanks go to Andrea and Martyn Edwards for an amazing photo shoot and creating my back cover photo. **www.andreaedwardsphotographyuk.co.uk**

There have been many wonderful people in my life who have helped me along my healing journey and the writing of this book. I would love to acknowledge you all individually, but there are just too many to mention - you all know who you are in your own special way. I would like to take this time to thank you all so very much for your continued support, friendship and love. You are all a very special part of my life's journey. Here's to making many more happy memories.

Michelle Townsend

Suggested Reading

Richard Bach, *Illusions, The Adventures of a Reluctant Messiah* (Arrow Books, 1998)

Richard Bach, *Jonathan Livingston Seagull* (Harper Element, 2003)

Rhonda Byrne, *The Secret* (Simon & Schuster, 2006)

Dr. Joe Dispenza, B*ecoming Supernatural* (Hay House, 2019)

Dr. Joe Dispenza, *Breaking the Habit of Being Yourself* (Hay House, 2012)

Dr. Joe Dispenza, *You Are the Placebo: Making Your Mind Matter* (London: Hay House, 2014)

Donna Eden, *Energy Medicine* (Piatkus, 2008)

Michael England, *Miracles Happen with One Good Thought Freedom Series Book 2* (CreateSpace, 2011)

Dr David R. Hamilton, *How Your Mind Can Heal Your Body* (Hay House, 2008)

Dr David R. Hamilton, *It's the Thought that Counts* (Hay House, 2008)

Louise Hay, *You Can Heal Your Life* (Hay House, 1984)

Abraham Hicks, *Ask and It Is Given* (Hay House, 2004)

David E. Jones, *The Awakening of Death* (Socciones, 2020)

Bruce H. Lipton, *The Biology of Belief* (Hay House, 2005)

Anita Moorjani, *Dying to Be Me* (Hay House, 2012)

Prentice Mulford, *Thoughts are Things* (United Holdings Group, 2011)

Dr. Joseph Murphy, *The Power of your Subconscious Mind* (Pocket Books, 2000)

John C. Parkin, *F**k It: The Ultimate Spiritual Way* (Hay House, 2007)

Jane Roberts, *Seth Speaks* (New World Library, 1994)

Eckhart Tolle, *A New Earth: Awakening to your Life's Purpose* (Penguin, 2005)

Eckhart Tolle, *The Power of NOW!* (New World Library, 1999)

Brian Weiss, *Many Lives, Many Masters* (Piatkus, 1994)

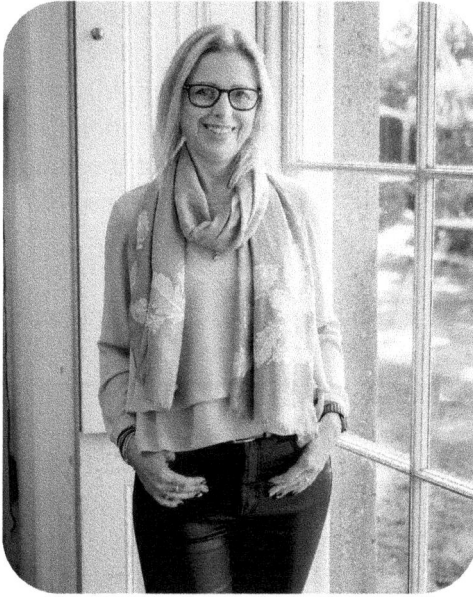

About the Author

Michelle Townsend was born and raised in Dudley, West Midlands, UK.

From a young age, Michelle always knew she wanted to be a teacher of music - teaching electronic organ, keyboard, piano and music theory. Running her music school for the last 37 years, Michelle continues to be a very successful music teacher, teaching all ages. Since Spring 2007, she has been the Dudley representative for London College of Music Exams, running practical and theory examination sessions for the area, which she continues to enjoy.

Michelle's choice to become a hypnotherapist in 2016 came after experiencing debilitating illnesses from Electromagnetic Hypersensitivity (EHS) and Hodgkin's Lymphoma Cancer.

After EHS peaked to its worst in 2007, Michelle sourced holistic therapies to help, turning to hypnotherapy and use of the mind. She started to experience relief from her symptoms but then, in 2010, was struck down again, being diagnosed with Hodgkin's Lymphoma, a blood cancer of the lymphatic system. Once again, she turned to hypnotherapy and the power of the mind/body connection.

Both journeys created powerful realisations and Michelle's life was transformed. Michelle has remained in remission for 14 years, now living a fulfilling life. She continues to enjoy working with private clients, helping cancer patients, running relaxation groups at a local cancer support centre, helping people with fatigue-related issues, and running talks and support groups in her role as a Certified Hypnotherapist. Michelle also achieved specialization in Hypno-Oncology in February 2022.

Michelle enjoys sharing her successes and inspiration to help others and is excited to add 'author' to the many accomplishments she has experienced in life.

www.harmonylifebalance.co.uk

www.ingramcontent.com/pod-product-compliance
Ingram Content Group UK Ltd.
Pitfield, Milton Keynes, MK11 3LW, UK
UKHW020720190325
456461UK00006B/396